NLP Dark Psychology:

Neuro-Linguistic Programming Techniques:

The essential guide To Persuade and Influence People, Learn to detect deception, covert manipulation and brainwashing behavior

J.R. Smith

Table of Contents

Introduction

What Is NLP?

Did you know that you can put a stop to your bad habits like smoking or eating junk food through hypnosis? Think about how much this could change your life and help you open the door to a more prosperous life! Did you know that you can learn many new and exciting things through NLP practices that may help you improve yourself and your life? Although you may have been unaware, there are many ways that you can use NLP methods to improve yourself and your experience!

Your first question may be, "What exactly is NLP or Neuro-Linguistic Programming?" You may have never even heard this term before, let alone know what it means and what it's all about! This is a fair and essential question! When learning about any new topic, it's vital to understand the foundations of it. This could not be truer for the issue of NLP as well!

Neuro-Linguistic Programming was created in the 1970s by a pair of self-help trainers in California. It is an approach that attempts to aid communication skills, psychotherapy, and personal development.

Based on the idea of this therapy, there is a connection between our brains (neuro), language (linguistic), and learned behavioral patterns (programming). It is believed these three things can be changed to alter and, hopefully, improve one's behavior or accomplish specific goals. The creators of this approach, as well as many others who practice or use it, claim that an entire slew of issues, problems, and obstacles in life can be solved through this self-help therapy. Depression, addictions, phobias, allergies, the common cold, or learning disorders are just a few that are believed to be treatable through this therapy. There have even been claims that some have been treated in as short as a single session!

There are also many different strategies and types of Neuro-Linguistic Programming, and in the coming chapters, we will explore how you can implement them into your life to make positive changes that will, hopefully, lead to outstanding personal success! A few of these strategies are hypnosis, memory alterations, and reframing. Although these may seem like very foreign and even strange concepts to you now, don't worry! This book will help you to explore many of the different NLP topics and help you to understand just what they are! Let's begin!

In this section, we are going to take some time to shift our focus and spend a bit of time looking at NLP. The idea of NLP, known as neuro-linguistic programming, was first developed by Richard Bandler and John Grinder in 1976. This is going to be comprised of three parts including the neuro that is going to focus on the neurology, the linguistics that will reference back to language, and then programming that will refer to the function of that neural language.

These men spent some of their time studying three individuals and their ability to change up the feelings and thoughts that they had. Over the years, many have adopted these ideas, although there is some criticism out there that looks at the legitimacy of the results of the study.

NLP is more of a thought, rather than a process, that can be used on other people. It is more of something that you should concentrate on yourself. The basic ideas that come with NLP are that you want to change the thoughts and the feelings that are inside yourself. Doing this is excellent for those who would like some relief from things like depression, anxiety, and some of the other mental illnesses that are out there. These individuals may feel that there is a specific thought or another belief that is holding them back, and when they can make changes to these things, the individual can change their life.

An excellent example of this would be when someone decides to make themselves believe that they like exercising, even if they disliked it ahead of time. Some people have found that using the tactics that come with NLP can bring them some success. But some have criticized the capabilities of this process and how well it can work for those who choose to use it.

There are going to be some benefits that come with neurolinguistics programming, no matter what side of the debate you are on, but there are some issues because it can be used as a tactic for manipulation. NLP intends to be able to look inward to figure out what makes the person unique and their person. The things that form the beliefs of that person are also going to indicate the quality of life they are going to have. The idea here is that by changing up these beliefs, it is easier for that person to change or improve different parts of their life.

Some manipulators will learn about the NLP ideas and then will use these in more dangerous manners. These manipulators are going to use some of the tactics that come with NLP to try and convince their victims to do things that may harm the victim, but which are going to benefit the manipulator in one way or another.

Now, you may be wondering how someone would be able to use the ideas of NLP to manipulate you. First, we need to take a look at what some of the tactics of NLP are, and then we can see that there are many ways that the manipulator can use this against you.

There is some positivity in this way of thinking, so even for those who don't find this in their lifestyle in the form of manipulation can find that practicing NLP, or at least learning more about how it works, will help them in different ways. Let's take a look at some of the parts that come with NLP in this section and why it can be such a powerful tool.

How We Receive Information

The world that we live in is going to be carted based entirely on what we decide to put our focus towards. What we choose to put all of our energy towards is going to help to build up the foundations for what we think, feel, love, express, work, and do. So basically, the things that we put our focus on is going to make us into the individual we are today, and it is the reason that we are so different from everyone else in our world.

We can see this just by looking at the different areas a person can live in. Someone who has always lived in California is going to see the world in a different way than someone who lives in rural Texas. These are both humans who live in the United States and may have been born there, they are going to have completely different lives, and this leads them to have different morals, beliefs, and perspectives. You are only going to notice what you tune your attention on, and not what other people do. Your world is going to be so different than the one that is going on around you. For example, it is possible that you would work at the same place for years and have no idea how many car dealerships are present on the route that you usually take to get to work. You may take the same streets to the same place for work, each day, every week, and for years at a time, and never realize that you go past three dealerships along the way.

Then, at some point in all of this, your car breaks down and instead of repairing it, you decide to purchase a new vehicle. Once buying a car becomes the goal for you, you may start to realize that there are that many car dealerships to check out. But before that time, the car dealerships were low on your attention, and you may not have even noticed. Oftentimes, this is why people will see signs. The signs that we think to point us in a specific direction is usually just going to be the mind looking for outside validation for something that we already want. For example, if you are considering whether or not it is time to have your first child, you may start to notice things around you that would relate to this. You may begin to notice how many baby commercials are on television, or notice that a woman is holding their baby on the boss. Seeing all these things may convince the person that they see signs and that it is time to have a baby.

In reality, you have just told the subconscious to become alert to all things about the baby so that you can pick up the signs that are around you, helping you to answer whether or not it is time to have a child. Since you alerted the brain that it is time to think about these things, and then it has become more aware of what is going on around it, and you are going to see things related to babies all around. It is incredible how much goes on around us. Because of this, the brain does block out quite a bit, or we would become overwhelmed in the process. We could go for years, maybe our whole lives, without realizing that there is something right in front of us. And then one day, we reach a trigger and then we are alerted to this thing and are surprised at how we never noticed it before, just like in the examples above.

Your Personality Profile

This personality profile is significant because it is what helps us to determine the information that we will store. Think about what are your hobbies, what are your interests, and what are your pet peeves. Think about what makes your skin crawl, what keeps you up at night, and what do you hope for in the future. These are some essential questions, ones that can make us unique individuals, and when they are all put together, they will make up our personality profile.

We all come with our agenda. No matter how much we wouldn't think of ourselves in this manner, and whether or not we are aware of it in the first place, there are always some motives or some reasons that we do what we do. For example, if you want to be wealthy, or at least have enough money to live off comfortably for some time, then you are going to look for more ways to make money and to save money. And for some people who want to have money but don't want to work, you may start to look for the best way to take advantage of other people and use manipulation to get what you want.

This goes to show that each person, no matter how pure their intentions, have a different reason, agenda, and motive for doing what they do. Your personality profile is going to determine how you will take in information and then what you end up doing with any of the information that you do take in. The primary forms of consumption, including your social media, television, and Internet consumption, can also take part in your personality profiles. The beliefs and the thoughts of your family and friends and what they share with you can contribute to the personality profile. And even the physical description of yourself, whether you are young or old, masculine or feminine, fit or fat, can all come together to contribute to what will be present in your personality profile as well.

The Animalistic Nature of the Brain

When we decide to take on some of the things that are around us, there are going to be some different questions that we may ask. For example, the first thing that we will often ask about some activity is whether it is safe or not. It is just instinctual for most people, even if they are not fully aware of it. The person may sense danger when it comes near, such as when they choose to not live in one area or another, or when they are near someone who makes them feel uncomfortable.

The next question that you may need to ask about here is whether the task has any value? Putting an amount on certain things will be different based on the person. You may value your job and your status in the work field the most while someone may value their family or their free time more. But even with these differences, there is some level of questioning about whether something is worth the effort or the risk when you make any decision. You also have to determine whether the thing is going to help you accomplish your goals. Even if it looks appealing, even if others recommend it to you, and also if it can do some things, if that tool, idea, relationship or job isn't meeting one of your needs, then it is not something that you should focus your attention on.

These wants and needs are going to be derivative of our biology. We may want more money so that we can purchase food or pay for our housing so that we can survive. Of course, this is a pretty obvious one. Another natural reaction of the brain, one that may be a bit subtler than the rest, is our desire to feel accepted and like we fit in. When we lived in a world, or our ancestors did, where forming these groups was necessary for the person to survive, we started to develop a natural urge to prove our worth.

In a typical tribe, there was a lot of roles that needed filled, and each person would be able to prove their worth by fitting into one of these roles. They would be the security, the gatherers, the nurturers, the hunters, and any other part that the tribe thought of as essential for the survival of everyone. Not everyone could be the hunter, but everyone would have their worth, and they would do what they had to prove their value and make sure they were able to stay with the tribe and survive.

We still have these kinds of desires, but they are going to be reflected in different ways. We always want to prove that we have some value, even though this isn't necessary for survival any longer. But we want to show this value so that other people are willing to keep us around. But some people in society will end up mistaking that. A woman could get some breast implants, or other work was done to prove that she is beautiful while putting too much value into her beauty and not on what makes her unique. The same can go for men.

A man may choose to sleep with many different women to prove their masculinity. When we can understand more about our natural biology—that urge that exists in everyone to prove that they have a lot of worth and should be a part of the group— it can be easier to start the process of redirecting our thoughts and changing the way that we look at the world.

Chapter 1: Neuro-Linguistic Programming and Mind Map

Now, we need to take a look at a new topic—the one of mapping out our reality. What everyone perceives is going to be completely different compared to what others see. A set of twins can end up with different outlooks on life. It is more likely that two people from different religious backgrounds and geographical backgrounds are going to come in with some different viewpoints. Still, those that are from places that seem similar might come in with different perspectives on what reality looks like for them, and this is often really surprising to a lot of people.

Social influences will play a significant part in how each is going to act and develop. The background of people in the community can affect everyone. For example, if all of the people in one neighborhood are from more affluent backgrounds, then they are going to have a similar perspective on things. And then these viewpoints would come together and help that area to grow and function in one way. Now, it can go the other way as well. If there is a specific area where more people participate in the crime, lifestyle will likely affect others around. It isn't right for each person, and you are always going to have some exceptions. However, the location is also going to play a significant role in the way that they think. Another thing that can change the reality that we see in our minds is our biological makeup. Someone with a family history of depression and anxiety will directly affect their personality and even the way that they interact with other those around them.

Biological influences beyond just the wiring of our brain play an essential part in the mapping of our reality as well. Beyond just mental genetics—like eye color, skin, hair, and more—you also need to look at the beliefs, thought processes, and personality of the person. Whether it is more about nurture or nature is going to be a debated topic. This is likely a great blend of both that vary from one person to another. The family that this person was born into, as well as the people around them, can all change the way that the person is going to act and think throughout all the stages of their lives.

Meaning Is Very Subjective

Since our realities are so different, meaning will become varied as well. Some people will think that their whole purpose in life is to serve a higher power, such as God. Others may look at this meaning and feel that they are supposed to find happiness. Then, there are lots of those who think that there isn't a meaning to life at all—and whether or not there is one correct answer is really up to debate. Our social upbringing, genetic biology, animalistic behaviors, and personality profiles will end up defining our meaning.

This is part of the problem with the viewpoint of our worlds. Meaning can be subjective because it can be altered at any one time. Someone can spend their whole lives believing in God, and then because something happens in their life, they decide that they are an atheist. The opposite can happen, of course. There are countless stories of people who think that they will never be able to gain their faith, but then they find it and become some of the most active believers out there.

While we are on the topic, religion is so tricky because no one was born believing one thing. They might have always felt an individual spirituality deep down, but the ideas that come with Christianity, Islam, and Buddhist were all things that were taught. Meaning is explained to us in a specific aspect, but we can also go through and create our meanings and definitions as well.

The meaning of life is sometimes not going to be defined clearly for every individual, but everyone has their ideas on what they think is most important in their life. If they don't, that ends up affecting how they feel and act as well. However, you will find that there is a power in knowing that even though you believe something right now, no matter how hard you believe in it, you have the freedom to change your mind at any time. There are a lot of people who don't realize that they have this kind of freedom, and they get themselves stuck in one thing for years and years.

Now, NLP practices helping everyone realize this kind of power inside themselves, the power that they can use to make some changes in their lives. With the right NLP practices, the individual can look inside, figure out what is wrong in their lives, and then make some changes on the perspective they have on anything. Some people will run into more challenges doing this for some people, but it is something that everyone can try.

Since meaning is something so subjective, it can be comfortable in some cases to alter what others think or how they perceive the world. Many people are lost in the ideas of what they believe that they find it easier to give up the effort required to sort things out and latch on to any insights that others send out to them. When the person isn't able to figure out the ideas on their own or sort through their reality, it is easier for a manipulator to get ahold of them, and this can be dangerous. Some of those who use the practices of NLP end up using them to take advantage of others, merely because they have learned how to plant different ideas in the brain.

They can find their victim and alter the feelings of others, giving what they're masking as a solution to the problem that the lost individual, or the victim, has. In reality, even though this looks like the manipulator is trying to help out and put the good of the victim in front, it is just a way for the manipulator to get what they want or get closer to one of their own goals.

We Are Capable of Changing Our Feelings

People can change their feelings at any time that they want. Whether they did some soul searching and decided to change, or someone gave them the idea or something else, we as humans have a lot of freedom to change the way that we think or feel about someone. This is sometimes a tactic of manipulation that is used to control and persuade other people.

For example, one person can go through their entire lives for not caring whether or not their sibling borrowed their clothes. Then, one day, they will get mad at the sibling for a different thing, and then they lose it over the sibling borrowing clothing. This is a small example of this tactic, but it can be seen in various relationships.

Many feelings can be severe for the individual to overcome, but certain people will take these things and see how far they can push them. As we get older, and our meaning and worldview start to change; it is natural to see how our feelings are going to change as well.

Now, you will find that people are going to change these feelings in different ways as well, not everyone is going to go through and change in the manner that we think they should. There are some of those who don't change or change just a little, and they go through their whole lives with the same feelings. But then some will make changes every week or more, and it is often hard to keep up with what is going on. For most people, it is usually something in between these two.

Humans like to have comfort, and they will seek it out, just like any other animals. They don't want to continually change their thoughts or some of their long-held beliefs because they are afraid of what is going to happen. This can sometimes lead to some behavior that is dangerous and destructive, and sometimes, this leads to some patterns that are unhealthy and will stunt the personal growth of the person.

Some people may find that it is easy to change their feelings, and some may realize that it is debilitating to attempt to think or change their thoughts in any way at all. Each person is going to be different, and you are going to see all ends of the spectrum. But that is the beauty of this kind of freedom. You get to choose when you change things. Sometimes, we hold onto the thoughts and beliefs too long, and this can make it hard to grow. But there is a chance that we will change, and that we will change for the better, and that is the beauty of working with NLP tactics.

Chapter 2: Understanding the Dark Triad

Just when you thought manipulation was bad enough, here comes an even darker side of psychology, known as the Dark Triad. The triad is made of up three very distinct, yet interrelated personality types—narcissism, psychopathy, and Machiavellianism. Why are these three referred to as the Dark Triad or the darker side of human psychology? It's because these three terms define the very tactics—manipulation, persuasion, and coercion—that some people resort to in order to get what they want.

The term Dark Triad certainly has a sinister ring to it, and it is a term that many psychologists and criminologists use as a defining predictor that signals criminal behavior in an individual. Let's take a closer look at the three personality traits that make up this trifecta:

Narcissism - The term stems from the Greek mythology about Narcissus, the hunter who fell in love with his reflection when he saw it in a pool of water that he drowned as a result. So consumed was he by himself that he couldn't focus on anything else. Those with narcissistic personality traits often display symptoms which include being boastful, selfish, and arrogant, thinking only of themselves and nothing else. Narcissistic individuals also lack empathy and are extremely sensitive (one might even say hypersensitive) to any form of criticism, because they can't bear the thought of being imperfect or flawed.

Machiavellianism - This term stems from Niccolò Machiavelli, a renowned diplomat, and politician who lived in 16th century Italy. Machiavelli became notorious when his book, The Prince, was published in 1513. This publication was interpreted as Machiavelli's endorsement of the deceit and cunning that takes place in diplomacy. Oftentimes, those who tend to display Machiavellianist tendencies occupy only their self-interest, and they are manipulative and duplicitous. These individuals lack both morality and emotion, and they are not for anything else except for what's going to be beneficial to them.

Psychopathy - Antisocial behavior, manipulative, volatile, hostile, a lack of remorse or empathy are traits which are associated with a psychopathic personality. Psychopathic and being a psychopath are two distinctly different traits, with the latter commonly associated with or directly linked to criminal violence.

In 2010, Dr. Peter Jonason who was at the time an assistant professor of psychology based at the University of Western Florida and Gregory Webster, his co-author and associate professor of psychology based at the University of Florida came up with what is now being referred to as the Dirty Dozen Scale.

Jonason and Webster developed this scale as a method of measuring the traits that the Dark Triad comprised of. Within the triad, these three personality traits tend to overlap at some point and are characterized by the degree of self-centeredness, exploitation, disagreeableness, and manipulation that takes place. Jonason, Webster, and their team of researchers were trying to determine if sadism could be captured within the laboratory.

They were also trying to discover if these sadistic personality measures could be used to predict behaviors beyond the already established standards that the Dark Triad consisted of. In a second and related study that was conducted, the results interestingly revealed how individuals who displayed a high tendency of sadism, narcissism and (or) psychopathy were willing to act aggressively against an innocent party when aggression proved to be the more comfortable choice. A sadist would show a tendency towards higher levels of attack when it became apparent that their "victim" and could not fight back, unlike other "darker personalities," it was the sadists who were willing to spend the additional energy and time needed if it meant that extra effort was going to give them a chance to hurt someone else. This was a huge revelation, considering that in the past, other research studies revealed that while psychopaths had no problems inflicting hurt on others, they were much more likely to do so only if it served a specific purpose. Narcissists, on the other hand, were far less likely to engage in aggression unless they felt that their ego was being threatened, while Machiavellians resorted to aggression only if they thought the benefits were sufficient to warrant such action, and only if it involved acceptably low risks to themselves.

The individuals who took part in this study were rated from a scale of 1 to 7, and they were given a score which ranged anywhere from 12 to 84. The higher a participant's score was, the higher the possibility that they were individuals with one of the Dark Triad personality traits. Covert manipulative tactics are everywhere we look, from social media to the commercials that we are exposed to, even the sales tactics were bombarded with when we try to make purchases in person. Even children resort to manipulative tactics from time to time, as they begin experimenting with the different ways that work to give them the autonomy they seek. These tactics are even used by the people you love and trust the most, and here are some examples of ordinary everyday individuals who might resort to dark psychology more so than others:

True Narcissists - This one goes without saying. Those diagnosed as narcissists especially tend to carry with them an inflated sense of their self-worth, which means they always have a need to validate this belief by making themselves superior to others around them. Narcissists harbor dreams of being adored and worshipped by the masses, and they will resort to all sorts of manipulative and unethical behavior to get the adoration they want.

True Sociopaths - Those diagnosed as sociopaths often appear intelligent and charming, but their downfall is impulsiveness. Since sociopaths tend to lack the ability to feel any kind of remorse, they take advantage of these dark personality tactics to build relationships which are superficial and not genuine since they're only doing it for their benefit.

The Selfish People - Anyone with a hidden agenda that benefits themselves before others have the potential to resort to these dark, manipulative tactics if the outcome for them is a win.

The Politicians - To get the votes that they need, and to get the masses to vote the way they want them too, politicians are guilty of resorting to dark tactics of persuasion as a means to serve their end.

The Lawyers - Some attorneys will stop at nothing if it means they get to win their case, even if it means they have to resort to dark tactics to do so.

The Salespeople - Just like attorneys and politicians, some salespeople can be so focused on nothing but making a sale that they have no qualms about resorting to manipulative tactics to coerce a buyer into doing what they want.

The Leaders - Not all leaders are there to inspire, and some rely on manipulation to get others to comply with their demands.

The Public Speakers - Not all public speakers can be trusted, and there are some out there who will resort to manipulation if it means there's an opportunity to sell more products to do so.

These are just some of the many examples out there of people who will resort to the more malevolent side of the human personality spectrum, and always for no one else's benefit but their own. German-Danish research conducted recently revealed that while psychopathy, Machiavellianism, and narcissism do make up the Dark Triad, other personality traits could fall within a similar spectrum.

Examples of these include egoism, spitefulness, and sadism to name just a few, and as the research revealed, these malevolent traits all share one common thing, which is that they have a "dark core." It is very likely that if you display any one of these tendencies, you're might tend to the others as well.

Sadists have been mentioned several times throughout this chapter because those with the Dark Triad tendencies harbor within them the potential to overlap into sadistic behavior. You might even have encountered a sadist in your life once or twice. Maybe they're still in your life now. If you know anyone who would purposefully cause another emotional harm and derive great pleasure from it, that's a sadist. What makes a sadist dangerous is that their actions can range from anywhere between petty and severe.

Some common examples of what sadistic behavior might look like include:

- Purposely portraying another person in an unflattering way or false manner with the intent to damage to their reputation

- Purposely repeating secrets which they know are meant to be private

- Purposely trying to get a colleague fired behind their back

- Purposely jeopardizing a colleague's reputation in their absence

- Purposely marginalizing a colleague, family member, friend, or even an acquaintance

- Purposely trying to cause harm to someone else's relationship

- Resorting to bullying or cyberbullying

- Resorting to the theft of intellectual, physical, or financial property

A skillful sadist will set these situations up so carefully that it becomes difficult to prove they were they guilty party involved. What makes it worse is that they will never own up to the responsibility or feel any remorse for the damage that they have inflicted. People may even be reluctant to believe the sadist is behind the chaos because of their charming and likable personalities.

A sadist will intentionally seek out to harm someone else because they believe that it is going to benefit them to do so. They might resort to these underhanded tactics whenever they feel envious or threatened by another, or even if they perceive someone else to be weaker and less likely to retaliate. In some cases, it may not be clear as to why the sadist has chosen to launch an attack on the victim. We don't often think - or want to believe - that the sadist could exist within our own immediate circle of connections, but they do, and they could be your parents, siblings, extended family members, spouse, friends and the people that you work with.

Here's an example of a scenario when a sadist might be lurking in your midst among your family. Let's say this person - John Smith - lost his job not too long ago, and he was struggling with frustration and anxiety because he was having a hard time trying to find another. John seeks comfort and support by talking to his brother about it but requests explicitly that his brother keep the information to himself. John's brother agrees. After some time, John gets an invite to his brother's house for a casual get together. Thinking nothing of it, John is then taken aback when several guests offer their sympathies over the fact that he had lost his job and couldn't land another.

Embarrassed, hurt and angry, John immediately knows that his brother was the one who leaked his secret since he hadn't confided in his troubles with anyone else. When John confronts his brother, later on, his brother denies any knowledge and "has no idea" what John is talking about. John's brother continues to adamantly deny the accusations, making John feel guilty for suspecting him as the guilty party. It takes John a while to realize that this is not the first time he and his brother have been engaged in the same situation in the past, where John's brother has been responsible for several incidences which cause John either hurt or embarrassment while denying any responsibility.

The sadist could be anyone, anywhere and they're always lurking undercover making you question your own sanity as they purposely inflict harm and hurt in your life and then denying any kind of responsibility for it.

The Dark Side of Manipulation

We know manipulators exist and that they're all around us, but who are these people exactly? What sort of personalities do they have? In a romantic relationship, they're the partner who is abusive and controlling, damaging not just the relationship the two of you have built but taken your self-esteem down right along with it. In a family dynamic, they're the family member who continually creates disharmony and chaos, or the one who always wants to be the center of attention. They could be the sister, brother, aunt, uncle, cousin, mother, or father who makes subtle remarks aimed at making everyone else around them feel inadequate or insecure.

The manipulator could be your next-door neighbor or friend who is spreading rumors and gossip, the one who enjoys pitting one person against the other and then standing back and watching the fight. At work, the manipulator could be that colleague who has a track record for being dishonest and unethical, willing to stoop as low as they can to get what they want and stepping on everyone else's toes on their way to the top. Out on the streets, the manipulators are the criminals and con-artists who rely on deception and distraction to swindle you out of your hard-earned cash, robbing you in broad daylight without you knowing it and them stealthily covering their tracks to avoid being detected.

The manipulator can come in any shape or form, sometimes in the kind of a person you least expect, and among the several things that a lot of these manipulators have in common is the fact that they suffer from some form of personality disorder that makes them who they are. In 1835, physician Dr. James Cowles Prichard proposed the term moral insanity to describe these individuals who, although not technically insane by today's standards, had very significant and distinguishing differences in their attitudes and the way they behaved when it came to morality, ethics, and their emotional reactions or responses to certain situations. Despite these apparent differences when compared to other individuals, those classified under moral insanity showed very little social or emotional distress over their behavior.

These individuals who had a personality disorder of some sort had a long history of emotional, personality, relationship, and behavioral difficulties that were very significantly different from that of their families or even culture. The behavior patterns exhibited were dysfunctional and intruded into just about every aspect of their life, which created problems in their emotional and personal ability to function, which likely contributes to their manipulative tendencies. Among the personality types that are more like to resort to manipulation include:

i. **The Histrionic Personality Type** - The individual with this pervasive behavior tends to seek out attention and resort to excessive displays of emotion, often referred to as being dramatic. When involved in a relationship, they can resort to highly manipulative behavior to get what they want.

ii. **The Antisocial Personality Types** - These individuals are capable of being manipulative because they hold little regard for the unspoken societal rules that everyone else follows. These antisocial personalities could consist of a range of behavior patterns, which include being unsupportive, chronically unreliable and irresponsible, conning others and for the ones who have no regard for another person's fundamental rights could even resort to criminal activity and show no remorse for it. Clinically, these individuals are incredibly selfish, with lying, deception, intimidation, and even physical assault being part of the many behavioral patterns they could potentially exhibit.

iii. **The Borderline Personality Disorder** - These individuals can be intense, volatile, and unstable when it comes to their self-perception, moods, and relationships. They have little to no ability to control their impulses, and the common characteristics associated with this type of behavior include fear of abandonment, being unstable when it comes to their self-image, social relationships, displaying inappropriate but intense feelings of anger and paranoia, and even resorting to impulsive or self-damaging acts which include substance and alcohol abuse. This instability could then lead them to perform actions of manipulation.

iv. **The Narcissistic Personality Disorder** - having a narcissistic personality is a disorder which leaves to a sense of entitlement, a need to be admired, and an inflated sense of self-worth. It is not uncommon for these individuals to have a huge ego, and they care little for anyone else but themselves. This lack of empathy for others, arrogance, inflated self-esteem, sense of entitlement which leads them to believe that they deserve to have special privileges and attention can lead towards feelings of jealousy or envy when their needs are not being met.

This high sense of entitlement also leads them to believe that they have a right to punish or exact revenge on anyone whom they perceive as not giving them the attention, due respect or admiration that they think they deserve. Psychologically, narcissism is not capable of genuine self-love, since those who struggle with narcissism are more in love with the comic and idealized, unrealistic image of themselves that they have built up in their minds.

These delusions of grandeur that they harbor within them are just what leads to such dysfunctional behavior, and why these individuals are more often than not described as demanding, selfish, condescending, and manipulative. Their friendships, family life, romantic relationships, and even professional relationships are not safe from their narcissistic tendencies, and what makes it harder is that those with this personality disorder are reluctant to change, preferring instead to expect others to conform to their needs.

Chapter 3: Manipulation and Behavior Conversion

The following chapter will discuss everything that you need to know about manipulation and mind control. Do you want to make sure that you can get others to agree with what you like? Are you interested in getting a better lifestyle, getting people to purchase something, and so much more? If so, then this guidebook is so fantastic, especially if you like to learn about manipulation and how it can help you out!

What Is Manipulation?

When it comes to manipulation, it seems that a lot of people underestimate how powerful it can be and frequently, they will misunderstand what is going on with this art form. It is common to see the word manipulation and believe automatically that the other person is trying to be emotionally abusive, mean, and cruel. We automatically associate a lot of negative traits back to the words.

While people can use manipulation negatively, it is essential to remember that there are some positive parts of manipulation as well. Because so many people see manipulation as a negative thing, it can prevent them from realizing just how powerful of a psychological art form manipulation can be. Furthermore, many people fail to understand that pretty much each of us already uses manipulation in one manner or another—just by living our day-to-day lives. While we may not automatically see this kind of behavior as manipulation, we all will have some degree of practice with using it.

Learning how to manipulate effectively doesn't mean that you are heading out into the world and trying to create some abusive patterns between yourself and those around you. Instead, it just means that you know what you want, and you have refined the method that you want to use to get it. When it is all said and done, if someone doesn't want to give in to what you want, they won't.

Manipulation isn't all about the pressure put on the other person. The best manipulators don't force someone into doing something that they don't want to do. Instead, it is more about helping someone see the value in helping you and doing what you would like and then building up from there. Before we start to look at some of the techniques that you can use with manipulation, we first need to dig deeper into what manipulation is all about, how and why manipulation tends to work, and when you would decide to work with manipulation in your own life.

To those who aren't fully aware of manipulation and what it is all about, it is hard to see that this process takes up three steps. Most of us will think of manipulation as one thing—there need to be two things in addition to the act of manipulation, which will make sure that the manipulation is successful. These include the analysis, which happens first; and the persuasion, which is going to take place for most of the conversation with the victim but is primarily going to show up after the manipulation. Understanding that there is more to the art of manipulation than just the act of manipulation itself is going to help you understand more about what can make the process more successful. While beginners may think that they can do it without the persuasion and the analysis aspects, you will quickly find that the results aren't as good if you miss these two parts and that you are less likely to get the things that you want.

Can Someone Use Our Map of Reality Against Us?

Once we can define our world, it is often easier to go through and pinpoint all of the things that tend to make your world unique. Some people will then start to exploit this kind of individuality in the hopes of trying to connect with you on a more personal level. For example, you may meet someone new, and they might be able to notice that you like henna tattoos, and in an attempt to get a bit closer to you, they go out and get one. But then you find out that they are doing this to get something from you.

This is an example of a manipulator. The manipulator has found a way to break into your world by disguising themselves as someone they can relate to. When in reality, when they are just trying to distract them from getting closer. There are times when people are going to come into your life to make you rethink your choices based upon your world. They might make you question whether this idea or this new person or the unique situation to fit in with your own beliefs? Are you sure that you are not going against anything you believe in? If you encounter an excellent manipulator, someone more of a master at it will make you question your morals, and then when your beliefs become vulnerable, they are going to swoop in and see whether or not they can take advantage of that.

Let's take a look at an example of this. If you know someone and they know that you are a somewhat religious person, they may try to manipulate you by using religion against you. They may be able to use that to their advantage and play on your weaknesses. They may know that as a religious person, breaking your moral code can end up causing a lot of pain. They can even use guilt and some of the other tactics of manipulation about the things that matter to you to make sure that they get what they want.

Mimicking Your Body Language

Hence, the first thing that we are going to take a look at here is the idea of the manipulator, and of those using NLP tactics, using mimicking body language to help them. Those who are good at handling these kinds of tactics will start to mimic the body language of the victim they are working on. This helps the victim feel like there is a closer connection with the manipulator, and they often don't even realize that it is happening.

Hence, if the victim is standing with their hand on their hip, then the NLP user is going to do the same thing. If the victim is overly confident, with their chest puffed out and their arms crossed a bit, then the NLP user is going to do the same thing. The point here is that the manipulator is going to pay close attention to their victim and the body language that the victim is using, and then they will copy that. This helps to form a connection between the victim and the manipulator, letting the victim know that the manipulator is someone they can trust and depend on.

In some cases, a masterful NLP manipulator is going to be able to start similarly talking to the victim. Hence, if someone is overly enthusiastic, the NLP user might feed on that enthusiasm, exerting a good mood and overall happiness as well. This can also go the opposite way in terms of personality. If the manipulator comes across someone who seems more pessimistic or someone who complains often and likes to share negative views, then the user of NLP is going to work on matching this and will send out the same kind of attitude in the process.

The manipulator may even use the sense of touch to their advantage, touching the other person a bit to form a stronger connection. This can be a bit violating, but some people are so thrown off by this kind of touch that they aren't able to notice that the manipulation is going on. This can often happen in the workplace, and even in a school setting. A teacher or a boss may come up behind the student or the worker, and then places a hand on their shoulder this can seem friendly in some cases, but it is often one of the ways that are used to exert power over the other person, or the victim. To make sure that the situation doesn't become uncomfortable, most people and most victims will allow the other person to touch them. While the victim was trying to avoid a scene, the manipulator was able to gain more power only by using the touch.

If you want to make sure that someone isn't mimicking your movements or trying to use NLP on you, try to do some strange things, things that you wouldn't usually do, and then check to see whether the other person is working on the same thing. Maybe you can find a funny trick that you can do with your hand, like tapping the top of your head lightly as you talk. You can move your eyes around rapidly, or tilt the head to the side back and forth.

If you do some things that are out of your norm, and you notice that the other person is doing them as well, then there is a high probability that they are trying to use some of the NLP tactics on you. This is the same idea that you can do for anyone who tries to touch you during a conversation or at work. If you don't feel like being affected by this person, don't stand by being quiet; take some time right then and there to call that person out. You don't have to make a big scene, but politely asking them to stop will usually get them to let up and not doing it again.

Now, it is essential to realize that some people will adopt the mannerisms and behaviors of those around them because that is how their personality is. This is more of codependency, rather than a tactic of manipulation. To figure out the true intentions of the other person, you may need to look at that person and figure out what they are likely to gain from the situation. If they don't seem to be taking anything from you as they do it, then this is a sign that it is behavior that is harmless.

Cold Reading

Another thing that can happen with NLP tactics is a process that is known as cold reading. This is when the manipulator is going to try and convince you that they already know more than they do. Some people who do this already include psychics, fortune tellers, mediums, and mentalists. They will use it to make the victim feel like the manipulator is more aware of specific facts. Those that know how to read cold can pick up on your verbal cues and your body language very quickly and can soon understand how you work and who you are. From there, they can use a series of guesses to figure out information, to analyze what they see in your body language, and other responses that the victim gives to learn whether they are right or not.

For example, a psychic could start with a group and tell these people that they are speaking with someone, and that person has a name that begins with J. Now, most people in the audience likely knows someone in their life who died and had a J name, so these people might assume the psychic is talking about someone they knew. The audience member may even speak up and say something like, "My uncle Jason just died." The supernatural will then go with that audience member, playing off their body language, and making some small, and very general guesses, that the member of the audience can relate to their own life.

Confusing Phrasing

Those who like to use the tactics of NLP are going to love gibberish. They will say some quick phrases, or they may hide certain words in bulky sentences so that they can sneak in the real meaning of what they would like to speak to the victim. This is something that we can regularly see in advertisements. Maybe there will be an overload of information. Listen to a commercial that has some medication or another being advertised. In this one, the whole business is going to talk about the medicine and how great it is, and then in the last little bit, usually just a few seconds, there will be a rapid reading that contains all of the cautions and the warnings that a patient should know about taking that pill.

This kind of thing can also be seen in the different types of interactions that we have with people. You will find that younger kid, and even teens can be useful for this. They may ask for permission to get or do something, and then they will start with all of the reasons why someone would say yes to the request. Then, in the end, they will rush through any of the reasons that the parent or another person would tell no to the application.

Someone who is using NLP is going to make sure that they stay pretty vague on what they say. They could go with jargon that is quick so that you can be distracted, or they will be so general that you become confused about the actual intentions because you can't stick with any of the words or thoughts. An excellent example of this is some of the political phrases that have become popular over the years. Obama used "Change' in his campaign, which is something that could appeal to anyone. This is something that many manipulators can use too. They will stick with sayings that are vague so that they can appease the most significant number of those around them.

These manipulators may say things like "I'll take care of it," and then they won't offer up any ideas or explanation of how they are going to fix that problem. Then, other manipulators might include those that leave out any information that might alter the perspective of the victim, and they will choose to stick with general information.

Using Your Wants Against You

The last thing that we are going to take a look at is the idea that manipulators and NLP experts are going to learn how to use your wants, or the desires of their chosen victim, against them. Those who are skilled in using NLP are easily able to tell and know what they want. This is because they have wants that are serious as well. While everyone has their individual and unique experiences, ones that can keep them apart from others, it isn't uncommon for many of us to share the goals. Achieving fame or fortune or reaching true happiness can be big ones.

You will find that those manipulators who are good at using NLP are practiced at knowing what people want. They can then use these desires against the victim to get what they want. Remember that the manipulator can feed off the emotions of their victim, and the manipulator isn't going to care how your feelings affect you, but how they can use these emotions against you. For example, they may be good at finding those who want more attention or seek the approval of others and then prey on them to get what they, the manipulator, wants.

Those who can use the tactics of NLP are going to be more dangerous than the manipulators who we talked about before. These individuals can take it a bit further, and they can take the time to study how the brain works, and then can use this to their advantage. If you feel that someone is using these tactics of NLP against you, then you may find that it is harder to deal with and avoid compared to regular manipulation, and often it is harder even to recognize. But the good news is that you can continue to use the same techniques that we talked about before, earlier in this guidebook, to deal with these kinds of manipulators as well.

NLP is a decorative technique that individuals can use on themselves if they are interested in learning more about themselves and making changes to the way that they think and view the world. But if these techniques are used in the hands of the manipulator, it can be a dangerous tool, one that is hard for the victim even to recognize, much less fight against.

How and Why Does Manipulation Work?

Despite what it may seem, manipulation is going to work efficiently. For the most part, people are going to be automatically wired to say no to something the first time that they hear about it. This happens if whoever is asking the question is someone the victim doesn't know or trust already when it is someone that the victim trusts, they are more likely to think about the subject and there is a higher odd of them saying yes.

Let's assume for a moment that you don't already know the other person and that you haven't been able to build up their trust before you work to manipulate them. As a result, any time that you ask the other person for something, they are just going to tell you no. The idea that comes with this one is pretty simple. We do not typically like to take things from people who we do not have trust in. It is sort of like taking candy from a stranger or letting a stranger do something for you that could potentially leave you vulnerable and exposed to some threat. These are things that we wouldn't do. When someone we don't really know or trust asks you for something, there is always going to be that natural inclination to say no to them because we don't have enough confidence and history with this person to know what the result isn't going to be devastating in one way or another for us in the end.

The same is going to be true of others when you try to manipulate them. If you ask someone for a favor, there is a high chance that they will also say no to you, unless you already know them and have built up trust with them. Of course, there are steps that you can take that can help you build up those feelings a bit quicker so that you can get that yes much faster. With some practice and a bit more knowledge about the different manipulation techniques, you will be able to manipulate others and get a yes from them in no time.

Bad Manipulation

There are a lot of different types of manipulation that are available throughout the world—and often, we are going to think about the wrong form of manipulation. This is because most of us have heard about manipulation from books, movies, and the news. These sources are just going to spend time talking about manipulation and all of the bad things that had happened when someone used manipulation. How many times, for example, have you turned on the television and heard about some group or cult who took advantage of someone, or maybe a smaller group of people, and gotten them to change their whole personalities and more? You may have heard about some people being willing to kill, attack, and do more, even though they were the calmest and most controlled person in the world before this all happens.

Now, this is a little extreme, but there are many times when the manipulation is going to be seen as a negative thing. When this happens, it usually is because the manipulator is looking to get what they want, to gain something, without caring what happens to the other person. They may even want the target to become dependent on them to ensure that they can come back and use that person as often as they would like.

The target in this situation is often going to be the one who is harmed or hurt in some manner. Whether harmed physically in the process or are just led to believe that isn't worth anything at all, you will find that it can be damaging to the target. The one person who is going to be able to benefit with this kind of manipulation is the manipulator.

When Would I Need to Manipulate Someone?

There are quite a few times when you would have the desire to manipulate someone else. One example of this is a salesperson who wants to make a sale. Through the use of some of the strategies we will talk about for manipulation, the salesperson would be able to develop any opportunities that are needed to easily and quickly establish a rapport. Once that rapport is set up, they will find that the sale with the victim, or the customer, in this case, is going to close quickly.

People are much less likely to give you the answer of no when they trust you, and you can get them to take the time to listen to your offer. This can also be true when it comes to making any recommendations as needed, requesting someone to help you, and pretty much any other time that you are trying to get your way. The idea is that if you would like to convince someone else to get what you want, you will make sure that you are never harmful to someone else in the process, you could use manipulation to help you get the thing that you want.

When Should I Avoid Manipulating Someone?

Despite all the power that can come with manipulation, there are going to be some times when you shouldn't use it at all. You will find that people can't be manipulated unless there is some willingness for this to happen. If you come across someone who is entirely against agreeing with you and doing what you are asking them to do, there is no way that you can go in and change their mind without calling on manipulation tactics that are often seen as abusive, cruel, and harsh.

If you want to master the art of manipulation, you must make sure that the delicate boundaries are kept, and that you work on the right strategies, without being harmful to the other person in the process. There are going to be times when the victim says no to you, and as the manipulator, you need to respect the no that they give. Of course, this doesn't mean that you have to give up completely, you could still call on some of the tactics of persuasion to see if you can organically get the other person to change their mind. However, you should not try to force the other person to change their mind or opinion. When you try to force your ideas on the other person, this is where the concept of manipulation starts to turn into a bad thing that needs to be avoided.

How Do I Spot Manipulation?

All of us want to make sure that our needs are getting met, but most of us are not going to rely on underhand methods to make this happen. A manipulator on the other side of things is more than happy to covertly influence someone with abusive tactics or indirect and deceptive tactics. There are many times that these manipulators may seem like they are courteous and friendly, and they can be good at flattery. They know how to make the other person feel important, but in reality, the manipulator only does this as a way to achieve their ulterior motives.

Manipulation can go the other way as well. Sometimes, they will lean more to using hostility and abuse to gain what they want. When this happens, the objective with that person is to gain power, more than trying to achieve anything else. In some cases, the victim won't even realize that they are being intimidated consciously.

There are a lot of weapons that a manipulator likes to use, and they are not afraid to bring as many of these out to help them as physically possible. They could use foot-in-the-door, reversals, evasiveness, sympathy, apologies, fake concern, comparing, denying, complaining, simulating that they are ignorant or innocent, and so much more.

If they can use a method to get what they want, no matter how underhand it may be, the manipulator isn't going to feel bad for using that to their advantage. Some manipulators are going to deny that they made specific promises, that certain agreements had been reached, or even that a conversation had ever occurred. They can also blame their victim for something that the victim didn't do so that they can gain power or sympathy. This is an approach that is used to break out of an agreement, promise, and date. You may even see a form of manipulation with parents who like to use bribery, such as "finish your dinner to get dessert."

Another thing that you can watch out for with manipulation is that the manipulator is often going to voice assumptions about your beliefs and intentions, and then they will react to these as if they were right. This is one of the ways that they can justify their actions or feelings. At the same time, they will continue to deny what the victim has said in the conversation. The manipulator may act as if something has been decided on or agreed upon when it hasn't, because this can help to put down any of the objections that you could have about that situation.

This small request is followed by real demand, and this one is usually a lot larger. The victim may find that it is harder to say no to this second request because they have already said yes to the other one. If the victim does try to say no to the second request, the manipulator is ready to jump in and act like the offended party. They will turn around the words of the victim quite a bit, and they will make sure that they are the one is hurt in this scenario, in the hopes of getting the victim to do what they want. They are very skilled at making sure that the situation is about them and their complaints, and that puts the victim on the defensive, even though they had been willing to help out with the original request.

Faking concern is another technique that a lot of manipulators are going to use to get what they want. This method is a good one because it can undermine the confidence and the decisions that come with the victim because the manipulator is willing to use warnings and worry about the victim.

Another thing that you can look for when it comes to manipulators is the idea of emotional blackmail. The manipulator could use guilt, shame, threats, intimidation, and rage to get the victim to do what they would like. Shaming can be used because it will create some self-doubt in the victim and could make them very insecure about what they have said or done. Oftentimes, the shame is going to be hidden in a type of compliment, such as saying, "I'm surprised that you of all people would stoop to that!" In some cases, the blackmailer is going to try and frighten their victim with anger, to force that victim to sacrifice their own needs and wants. If this doesn't end up working for them, the manipulator could switch from being frightening to being angry. The victim will notice the change and will feel so relieved at the difference that they will agree to do whatever the manipulator wants.

You can also watch out for what is known as passive-aggressive behavior. When you have trouble saying no to the other person, you may agree to things that you don't want to do—and then you can still get your way by forgetting, being late, or doing it halfheartedly. In most cases, passive aggression is going to be a way for you or the manipulator to express hostility. Forgetting on purpose can help you to conveniently avoid the thing that you didn't want to do in the first place, and enables you to get back at your partner.

Of course, sometimes, we do this without realizing it. Maybe we do forget to do something because we don't hold it as necessary enough to remember. Sometimes, it happens without meaning to hurt the other person we don't want to do it. However, the manipulator is going to take it a bit further and will try to get the other person to do what they want, or will get out of something that they don't want to do, by conveniently forgetting or not doing the work the way that they should.

As you can see, manipulators are going to come in all sorts of shapes and sizes. It is hard to know for sure whether you are dealing with a manipulator or not because they often can use many faces, and often, you are pretty close to them from the start. A manipulator isn't going to be someone who randomly comes into your life one day. You already know that these brand new people need to build up your trust, and that can take some time. For the most part, when you are being manipulated, it is going to be by the people who are close to you, a friend, family, or even a coworker.

Learning the signs of manipulation, and asking yourself the right questions to see whether manipulation may be going on can be the first steps to take to help protect yourself. If you know what is going on and can speak out about it from the beginning, you will find that it is easier to avoid the manipulator. Manipulators want to get what matters to them. If the other person is putting up a big fight or has caught on to what the manipulator is doing, then the manipulator is going to find someone else.

Some Examples of Manipulation We Can Find in Our Day-To-Day Lives

Manipulation is all around us. There are so many people in our daily lives who are looking to manipulate and convince others to go along with what they want to the point that it can feel like everyone is out to get the others. There are a few situations where manipulation can become more apparent, and when you look through a few of them, you may start to realize that you have already dealt, or are currently dealing with, a few of these examples below:

Home-Court Advantage

Someone who is trying to manipulate another person is always going to try and gain the upper hand in the situation. They may find that it is easier to invite their victim to a meeting, or to interact in another way, in a physical space where the manipulator will be able to exercise more control and dominance. The manipulator may choose to meet with their victim to discuss something in the car, office, home, or in some other space where they feel more ownership and familiarity, while the victim may not be familiar with these at all.

The victim will usually agree to meet in this place because they think that the manipulator is friendly and hospitable. This allows the manipulator to have the upper hand that they are looking for, but the victim is not going to realize that this is what is going on until it is too late.

Allowing You to Speak First

Many manipulators like to acknowledge their victim to speak first. This can work in several ways. First, the victim is going to leave with the false sense that they were the ones in charge. Also, they might think that the manipulator was deferring back to them, but in reality, the manipulator likes to let their victim speak first so that they can get a baseline for where the victim is, sniff out any of the weaknesses, and then uses this to their advantage along the way.

This is something that you will see with sales quite a bit. The salespeople will ask their victim some general and probing questions. This allows them to establish the baseline of the victim's behavior and thinking. From here, they can get a good idea of your weaknesses and strengths. This type of questioning will have a hidden agenda, and we may be able to find it in other places of our lives, such as in personal relationships and the workplace.

Changing Around the Facts

If the manipulator can change up some of the facts that are present in the discussion, they are going to do so. They are primarily going to do this if they find that changing up the circumstances will put them in a better light. There are a lot of examples of this that we can see in our day-to-day lives. They may show a one-sided bias of the issues, or work with exaggeration. Sometimes, the manipulator will strategically withhold information that is key to the victim, making the right decision. They may try to blame the victim for causing their victimization; they may deform the truth; they may lie and make excuses up as well.

Adding in Lots of Statistics and Facts

Some manipulators like to use the idea of intellectual bullying against their victim. This is done when the manipulator presumes to be the expert and the one who is the most knowledgeable in certain areas. The manipulator is going to be able to accomplish this technique by taking advantage of their victim using alleged facts, statistics, and some other data, especially if this information is stuff that the victim may not know much about.

We may see this kind of tactic when we are looking at financial and sales situations. In these, the professional is going to presume that they have the expert power over you, and they hope that because of this, they will be able to push through their agenda onto you easier. Some people like to use this kind of technique just for the benefit of feeling a sense of intellectual superiority over other people.

Overwhelming You with Red Tape

In some cases, the manipulator is going to work to overcome their victims with the use of a lot of red tapes and a lot of procedures. This is a tactic that is known as bureaucracy. This is going to include a lot of laws and by-laws, systems, paperwork, committees, and a ton of other roadblocks that are put in place solely for the idea of making the life of the victim more difficult. In addition to helping the manipulator have the upper hand over their victim, the manipulator could use this technique to delay any truth-seeking and fact-finding. It is an excellent way to distract the victim who may be catching on to the manipulator, and it can help hide the weaknesses and flaws of the manipulator while ensuring that they can evade scrutiny as much as possible.

Raising Their Voice to Showcase the Negative Emotions

The next thing that the manipulator could do is raise their voices to make sure that the victim knows that they are going through negative emotion. This can often happen during a discussion to showcase a form of aggressive manipulation. The assumption of the manipulator here is that if they project their voice and make it loud enough, or if they display enough negative emotions, the victim is more likely to submit and give the manipulator what they want.

Along with the loud and aggressive voice, the manipulator is often going to work on their body language to get the message across a bit more. They will make sure that their body language is active, such as standing tall or using a lot of gestures that show anger, excitement, and more to increase the impact of what they are saying.

Surprises That Are Done in a Negative Manner

Some manipulators like to work with surprises that are considered harmful to put their victims off balance, and because it allows them to gain the psychological advantage. There are several ways that the manipulator can do this. They could low ball during a situation of negotiations, or the manipulator could have a sudden profession that they won't be able to come through and do the thing that they had promised before.

In most cases, the unexpected negative information is going to come to the victim without any warning. This makes it hard for the victim to prepare and try to counter the move in the way that they would like. In the end, the manipulator could ask for some additional concessions from their victim to continue working together.

Limiting the Amount of Time to Decide

One technique that can be useful for a manipulator is to limit the amount of time that the other person gets to make a decision. When the victim feels like they are limited to time, they are more likely to go along with what the manipulator wants, even though not sure about the decision and they were not provided enough time to think it all through, and this is what the manipulator wants to see happening.

The idea of giving the victim little time to decide on things is a collective negotiation and sales tactic. This is where the manipulator is going to put some pressure on the other person to make up their decision, often before the victim is ready to make that decision. When you apply the tension and the control over the other person, the hope is that they are going to crack and then they will give in to the demands of the aggressor.

Poking at Your Weaknesses

Some manipulators are fond of making critical remarks, but then will disguise these remarks as sarcasm and humor. They can do this to make their victim feel inferior and less secure, but the fun helps the manipulator to save face and look better when the victim starts to get offended. In the process, they can make the victim seem less secure and inferior.

There are a lot of examples that come to mind with this one. The manipulator can have comments that will range from your personal belongings, your credentials and background, your appearance, and the fact that you came into the office just a few minutes late and seemed to be out of breath. The manipulator likes to point out the things that you did wrong so that they can impose their psychological superiority over the victim.

Criticism and Judgment Against You

This behavior is going to be distinct from some of the other practices that we have discussed. In those, humor was a kind of cover that the manipulator could use to say what they want, and then turn it back against the victim. However, with this one, the manipulator is doing away with the joking and is outright just picking on their victim.

By continually marginalizing, ridiculing, and dismissing their victim, the manipulator can keep their victim off-balance, while also making sure that they, the manipulator, can maintain their superiority. The aggressor would use this tactic to deliberately foster the impression that there is something always wrong with their victim, and that no matter how hard the victim tries, they are going to be inadequate and never good enough to meet the standards of the manipulator.

The thing here is that the manipulator only wants to focus on the negative and the bad things that go on. With regular criticism, there may be some bad things that come up in the discussion, but the other person is going to provide some feedback and some solutions that the victim can work on. With manipulation, the manipulator is just going to focus on the negative without giving any constructive or genuine solutions, and they never offer any meaningful ways to help the other person. They like to say and do things that will make the other person feel bad.

Using the Silent Treatment

We are all guilty of using this one at some point. We will get mad at someone, or feel that they slighted us in some manner, and we will stop talking to them. We think that we are making them suffer some when we don't give them our attention all the time and that by making them sweat it out for a bit, we are more likely to get what we would like.

Many manipulators are going to use this tactic as well. By deliberately not responding to the reasonable emails, text messages, calls, and other communications from the victim, the manipulator is going to presume the power. They are making the victim do all of the work, and this can place some uncertainty and doubt into the mind of the other person. The silent game is a head game, where the manipulator can use silence as a form of leverage against the victim.

Pretending to Be Ignorant of What They Are Doing

The next type of manipulation that you may run against is what is known as feign ignorance. This is pretty much the game of playing dumb. When the manipulator pretends that they don't understand what their victim wants, or what the victim would like the manipulator to do, the manipulator will then make their victim take on what is their responsibility and can make the victim break a sweat a bit.

There are a lot of examples of this kind of behavior in our modern world. Sometimes, we will see children using this tactic when they want to delay, stall, and manipulate adults into doing for them what they aren't interested in doing, such as cleaning their rooms. We can also see this kind of tactic in adults as well. Sometimes, grownups are going to use this kind of behavior or tactic when they are trying to hide some information, or if there is some obligation or task that they are trying to avoid doing.

Guilt-Baiting

The manipulator may choose to work with guilt baiting to target the vulnerabilities and emotional weaknesses of the target. The manipulator can do this to coerce the recipient of giving in and agreeing to demands and requests that are pretty unreasonable. Several examples can come up when you are trying to use guilt baiting as a type of manipulation technique. This could include holding the victim responsible for the success and happiness of the manipulator or holding the victim accountable for the failures and unhappiness of the manipulator. The manipulator may also rely on targeting the victims' soft spot and unreasonable blaming.

Victimhood

There are a lot of different examples of victimhood that can come from a manipulator. This could be things like the person playing that they are the martyr, powerless, and weak. They could try to deliberately be frail so that they get more favor and sympathy from those around them. Sometimes, there are thought of or exaggerated health issues, along with imagined or exaggerated personal matters.

The purpose of this kind of behavior is to exploit the goodwill of the recipient. It can also utilize the sense of obligation and duty, the guilt, and the protective and the nurturing instinct of the other person to get concessions and benefits that are unreasonable and that the victim likely wouldn't give to other people who weren't in the same kind of situation.

Modern Advertising

Often advertising is seen more as a form of persuasion compared to just being a form of manipulation but sometimes, it can be both. There are many well-known advertisers out there who will focus on using manipulation techniques to help them get what they want out of the other person. They can use foot-in-the-door, which shows you what other people want the product and more.

Many of us like to think that we are too smart to fall for the manipulation that is in commercials, online, and more, but as time goes on, many marketers are becoming even better at their jobs. They are supposed to convince you to go and purchase one product over another, or also to buy the product when you don't need it. If they are successful, you will part with your money to get the product, and the company can make some profits.

Even if we think that we can't be manipulated by advertising, this isn't true. Any a time that you go to the store and purchase a particular product over another, there is at least a partial inclination to do so because of advertisements that you saw. Sure, you may pick it for the price, or because it tastes good, or because it looks good on you as well, but at least, a small part of your decision was because of some advertising that you saw in the past.

As you can see, there are many different examples of manipulation that can show up in your day-to-day life. Depending on the people you spend your time with, you may find that there are a lot of different types of manipulation that could show up in your life. Learning what these are, and how to use them, can also ensure that you can get the results that you want when you are trying to manipulate someone else.

What Are Some of the Advantages of Using Manipulation?

Manipulation has been given a bad reputation. Frequently, we hear about manipulation in a lousy way, understanding that it is going to harm the target or cause issues for others, while the manipulator gets to run off and enjoy what they want and in some cases, this is just what manipulation is all about.

However, there are also times when the process of manipulation can be a good thing. A salesperson trying to sell a car to their target is making sure that the goal gets the vehicle that they want. A family member who is trying to get their child into therapy after a drug addiction may use manipulation to get them the treatment and the help that they need. Moreover, if you have ever heard a spiel about a fundraiser or a good cause, there are going to be some forms of manipulation present there as well.

There can be several valuable benefits that come from using manipulation. Whether you are working with manipulation in a good or evil manner, you will find that the manipulator and sometimes, the target can see a bunch of advantages in the process. Some of the benefits of using manipulation include:

Can Help You to Get What You Want

The main reason that people like to work with the idea and the process of manipulation is the fact that it allows the user to get what they want. In a world that there are wants other than time, knowing that you can walk into any room and talk to any person you wish to, and get them to agree with you or do what you want, can make a big difference. It is an enticing thing that many people are interested in learning more about, but few can learn how to make it all happen. It doesn't matter what you want to get out of someone else manipulation is going to help you to get there. Whether your intentions are good or not, manipulation can help you out. You could want the other person to help you out with a project or grab something for you for lunch when you are too busy to leave the office, or it could be something much bigger. Manipulation is going to be able to help you to get what you want.

Can Make You More Confident

You may find that working with manipulation is a great way to help yourself gain some more confidence. Many times we give up the things that we want because we are too shy, or we are too worried about what others think about us. We may even be worried that the other person is going to say no to us, and we aren't sure what we are going to do once the other person does tell us no about something.

However, when you are working with manipulation, you will learn the right techniques that are needed to make sure that you get what you want. You will learn the things that you need to say and do to ensure that your target will always agree with you. Think of how much this can help build up your confidence if you know that you can walk into any room and get the other person to agree with you, no matter what you ask.

Can Help You Get in the Relationship That You Want

There are times when you will be able to use manipulation to get someone to go out on a date with you and to ensure that you can get into the relationship that you are looking for. For those who have had trouble and some struggles with finding someone to go out with them in the past, this could be some welcome news. It may be that you need a little bit of confidence and a bit of communication, and you are set to get someone to go out with you.

You don't have to make this something that is sneaky or evil. Plus, that is not going to be the best way to get a new relationship up and going. However, you can use some of the techniques that we will talk about in this guidebook to help you to get that relationship going.

For example, if there is someone who you are interested in, you can use a few different techniques. Maybe you start to spend more time with them in an intellectual setting so that you can get more comfortable with each other, and learn more about what they like and dislike. This can help you to tailor your message to work the best for the personality of that person.

Another option to work with is the foot in the door method. This is where you would get them used to a bunch of small requests first so that they get in the habit of saying yes to you. You could ask them for help with a project, ask them if they think that you are a dependable person, and then slowly lead into asking them if they would be willing to go out with you. After they have spent some time getting that person to say yes to you, once you bring out that big request, they are more likely to agree, and you can get the date that you want.

Can Benefit the Other Person

If you are correctly using manipulation, you will find that it not only benefits you, but it can help the target as well. There are two main types of manipulation, and some of these are just going to benefit the manipulator, and others are going to be able to help all of the parties that are involved.

For the first group, the manipulator is just going to work on gaining their benefits.

They don't care what happens to the target. The manipulator may be just fine taking advantage of the target, and even causing them harm, as long as the manipulator can get what they want out of the situation. This can be hard on the target. Oftentimes, they will take years of abuse and mistreatment because they don't even realize that the manipulator is in their lives.

In these situations, the manipulator has made it so that the target feels they have no choice but to go with the manipulator. There is a codependent relationship going on here, and the objective is more than willing to agree to what the manipulator wants, even though it may not be the best for them. It can take a lot of work to get out of this situation, and it can go on for many years before any changes.

In the second situation, the manipulator is a bit nicer. They aren't going to focus so much on only getting what they want, although this is a part of the endeavor. The manipulator will be able to get what they want, but the target is going to be able to get what they want in the situation as well. The objective is not going to get harmed in this situation—and the manipulator is going to try to do something that will benefit and help out the target.

An excellent example of this is a salesperson. If the target goes out to get a car, they are going to deal with a little manipulation in the process. The salesperson will want you to go with a particular brand or type of car, or maybe the most expensive vehicle that they can because this helps them to get more back in commission. They will push what they want at the target, and the target can decide if they're going to get the vehicle.

Can Help Out a Certain Cause

There are times when manipulation is used in a manner that can help out a particular cause. If you have ever received an email or seen a commercial for some specific reason or fundraiser, then you have seen this in work. With all of the different types of charities and fundraisers out there, these organizations need to be able to convince you that it is best to spend your money with them, rather than with someone else and because of this, they are going to use a lot of manipulation on those who see their message.

No matter which organization you go with, and even though the organization is using some manipulation against you, it is still going to help someone else. The money is going to help some individual, animal, or another group that needs help—and this can end up benefiting everyone. The organization can help, those who need the help get the assistance that they need, and you get a feeling of doing something right and even a tax break at the end of the year if you choose to do it.

Can Help a Business to Make Some Money

One of the most significant places where we see manipulation in our day-to-day lives is from advertisements. There are thousands of companies in our country, and each of them is trying to work and get your attention, and convince you to spend your hard-earned money on their products, rather than spending that money on something else. In any of the advertisements that you have seen in your life, whether they are on the radio, on a website, on social media, print, billboards or somewhere else, you know some form of manipulation in place. Companies know that they need to be able to use manipulation against the other person, or their target audience, to get them to make the purchase.

The Negatives of Manipulation

Even though there are a lot of benefits that come with using manipulation, there are also some negatives that can show up as well. Unless you have a lot of experience working with manipulation, things could likely go wrong. The first issue is that manipulation can backfire, and often in a big way.

Many people can sense when they are being manipulated, and once they sense it, it can bring out a lot of resentment. If someone thinks you are trying to manipulate them, exert power over them in a sneaky way. Likely, that person isn't going to trust you in the future, and if you were successful at manipulating that person, even if they aren't begrudging about giving you what you wanted, they might start to withhold something from you to make sure they get even.

It is even possible that the manipulation is going to turn into a power struggle. Your target won't like it if they find out you have been playing with their feelings. Once they start to feel like that is what is going on, the power struggle is going to escalate, and trust can go right out the window.

Another issue is that we will sometimes try to manipulate others before we even think. Before we even know what we want, or before we also evaluate the possibility of asking for it directly, we may habitually go right towards manipulation. This can sometimes lead to the assumptions that can destroy the relationship that you have.

There are a lot of forms of manipulation that can become habitual when we are in a relationship. These can include guilt-tripping, abusive criticism, and complaining, to name a few. Another layer to all of this power struggle is going to develop, even if we didn't intend this to happen in the beginning and this all happens because we become too casual about our use of intimidation, emotional blackmail, and manipulation.

Besides, the manipulation isn't always going to be enough to satisfy. If you got someone to do something because of manipulation, how do you know it is something that they wanted to do or not. For example, if you bought a car because of a sneaky sales pitch, is there still a chance that you will purchase another vehicle. If the manipulator got what they wanted, but the price was a sense of secrecy and mistrust, is that want the manipulator wished to?

It can be tempting to use manipulation to get what you want. It seems an easy way to get what you want out of the other person, without using a lot of time working on trying to do the work on your own. You won't need to convince the other person to say yes but in the long run, if it doesn't end up benefiting the target, or it doesn't make sense for others to help you, then it isn't the best option for you to choose to go with. Some people are going to find that working with manipulation can work well for them. They may be able to perfect this kind of process and can get others to do what they want, without a lot of issues along the way, but for most people, this could end up being disastrous if they are not careful. You have to learn the right techniques to use to make sure that this is a successful endeavor and gets you what you want out of life.

Chapter 4: Simple Mind Control Techniques to Use

While we will take a look at some of the manipulation techniques that you can choose to use on your target, we are going to start with some of the methods that you can use with the idea of mind control. Mind control is a more intense version of manipulation, where the manipulator is going not just to influence the thoughts and decisions of the target but also to control every aspect of that target—whether it is their thoughts, actions, or feelings.

In this chapter, we are going to talk about some of the real mind control techniques that were traditionally used not just by ordinary people in interpersonal relationships but also in a group. Understanding how these work can help you either to use them if you need to influence the other person or to be aware of the manipulation that could be done against you. Some of the most common techniques of mind control that can be used will include:

Isolation

The first technique that can be used in mind control includes isolation. Humans are very social creatures. They like to spend some time talking with others, spending time out in public, having close friends, and family, and spending their time in more social situations. When we take this social aspect away from many individuals, it can change the way that they look at life.

Complete physical isolation can be the most powerful. This is when the subject is taken away from all contact with others, including email, social media, phone calls, and physical contact. This is something that has been seen in cults and with other groups. They will often take the person far away from others, and then the only human contact that the person can have is with the captors.

Now, this total physical isolation can be tough to do, and it is usually only done in really intense situations. If you are trying to use manipulation, you typically don't want to go through and completely isolate the target—but it is common for a manipulator will usually try to attempt their destination mentally as much as possible.

There are several methods that the manipulator can use to get what they want with the help of manipulation. They could include some seminars that last a week in the country and isolate the person from what they would usually do. They could be a lot of criticisms of the person's family and close friends so that the target feels bad and stops seeing them. It could be jealousy that keeps the target at home and limits the amount of influence that anyone outside the manipulator has on the person.

Once the manipulator can control the information that goes to the target, they can share information, withhold information, and do anything that they would like to continue influencing the target as much as they would like. The objective is going to become reliant on the manipulator, and this is how the manipulator can work and get what they want from the target. There are no outside influences to tell the target that something is wrong, or that they should watch out, and this traps the goal even more.

Peer Pressure and Social Proof

All of us like to feel like we can belong in a group. Some are centered on the idea of fitting in, and they strive to do everything that they can to be the life of the party, or to be liked, and so much more. Also, introverts spend more time at home rather than going out and partying and socializing all of the time, like to make sure that others like them, and that they fit in.

A manipulator can work to use peer pressure and social proof against you. They know where you tick when it comes to fitting in and getting others to get along with you. They will convince their target to do something because others do it, or because it is the best way to help you to fit in. Whether or not it is true, it is likely that the target is going to agree to it and will go along with what the manipulator wants.

Those who want to manipulate a bigger group of people, such as those who want to get others to donate in their cause, are typically going to use social proof, and even some form of peer pressure, to brainwash the newcomers. You will find that social proof is a phenomenon where some people assume that the actions and beliefs of others are appropriate—and they understand that because everyone else is doing it, then the effects are justified.

It often doesn't matter what the other action is at all. This is why we see a lot of people participate in activities that may not be regarded as acceptable in society once they get in with a group. This can work well when the individual is already uncertain about what they should think, how they should behave, or what they need to do. When people enter into these situations, they are going to take a look at what others around them are doing, and then choose to do those same actions, no matter what they are.

The manipulator can use this to their advantage. If they find a new target to work with, they will need to either implement them into a group of others who have been manipulated by that same person or try to convince the target that everyone else is doing the activity. Only by using this social proof and some peer pressure if others are involved, the target is more likely to go through and do what the manipulator wants.

Criticism

Criticism is used as a tool for isolation, but there are times when it can be used all on its own. Manipulators like to use criticism because it can make the other person feel insecure and like they are doing something wrong. The objection can be on a lot of different topics, from the clothes the person wears, how they look, who their friends are, and even their beliefs.

When a manipulator is trying to work with criticism, they often like to mask it behind a compliment or make it sound nice, with a little jab at the end. This allows them to use the criticism, but then fall back on the idea that the other person, their target, is just being sensitive or misheard them if the target becomes upset about the criticism.

Usually, the criticism is going to start pretty small. The manipulator won't want to start with something big because no one likes to be criticized, and if you start with something big, you will find that the target will just run off and not be around you any longer. The manipulator knows how to make comments that sound just a little bit hurtful and can plant a seed of self-doubt but which aren't huge or even that noticeable.

They could start with something like, "I didn't know that green was your color. I think you should ditch it." This one says that you don't look good in that color and can make fun of the clothes that the target is wearing. They may even choose to say something like this when you got dressed up and excited for a night out, or when you are wearing your favorite outfit. There wasn't necessarily anything mean about the thing that they said—but it was enough to plant some self-doubt in the person, especially given the tone and the situation at hand.

Over time, the manipulator is going to start making more obvious criticisms, to place some more self-doubt in the minds of the individuals they are directed at. This can make the target more reliant on the manipulator, because they start to feel like there are so many flaws in themselves, and that no one likes them. They see the fact that the manipulator is still near them as a sign that the manipulator cares, and they will start to do more and more that the manipulator wants in appreciation.

The manipulator may choose to criticize the outside world so that they have a better chance of claiming their superiority. According to the manipulator, you should feel so lucky that they choose to associate themselves with you. They make themselves seem important so that they can convince you that they are essential, and you should feel great that they want to spend time with you.

Forming a New Identity

This is one that is more likely to occur during the more extreme forms of manipulation, but it is still something that we need to take a look at. In some situations, the manipulator is going to try and redefine the identity of their target. This is going to ensure that they can get more of what they want out of the person. If they can get the aim to give up their old way of thinking and doing things, and end up with a blank slate, they can go through and fill in that blank slate with anything that they want.

In this case, the manipulator wants the target to stop being themselves, and they want them to become a robot, someone who is willing just mindlessly to follow their orders. Using all of the methods and the different techniques of mind manipulation that we have talked about in this guidebook, the manipulator is going to try and extract a confession from the target, some kind of acknowledgment that the target believes the manipulator is a right person and doing a good thing. Of course, there can be some slight variations to this, but it is pretty much the same idea no matter how this form is used.

At the beginning of this technique, it may be something that seems pretty insignificant. The manipulator may be trying to get the target to agree that the other members of the group are fun and loving people. It could be the manipulator trying to get the target to admit that at least some of the manipulator's views are valid. This may seem like a pretty simple thing to work with, but it is priming the target to start thinking with and agreeing with the manipulator on some items.

Once they can get the target to agree with them on some of the little things, it is much easier to get them to move on to some of the bigger things. Before you know it, out of the desire to be consistent with what you do and say, you would then find that the target starts to identify themselves as one of the group.

This is something that is going to take place in the long term. It is impossible to change the whole personality of someone in just a few weeks even. This can sometimes take a few years or more to happen. The manipulator knows that if they try to push the ideas on their target too quickly, the target is going to run away because they know what is happening. However, when they are brought into the group slowly and given time to think about it and learn more about it, they will find less resistance in the long run.

This idea can be compelling if the target knows that their confessions were filmed or recorded. Many manipulators are willing to record some of the things that their targets do and say. This allows them to have physical evidence to use against the target if the time comes. This may be a form of blackmail, but it is an effective way to make sure that the individual can stay in their place when it is needed. Besides, if the target ever forgets, this physical proof is going to show the new identity and shows the individual who they are now.

Repetition

The more that we hear about something, the more likely it is going to stick. This is one of the methods of mind control that a manipulator can use to their advantage if they keep repeating their message and using the same tools on their intended target to get what they want.

Constant repetition is another powerful persuasion tool. Although it may seem like a simple tool, easy to be effective, the act of repeating the same message as much as possible will ensure that the word is familiar and more comfortable for the target to work with. When the repetition combined with some social proof, it is going to ensure that the message is delivered without fail and that the manipulator can get what they want.

The existence of affirmations, which is a technique that is used in self-improvement, is another proof about how well repetition can work. If you can persuade yourself to believe or do something through repetition, then think about how easy it can be for someone else to use repetition to manipulate you to think and behave in a certain way as well. This method may seem simple to work with, but it is valid and will provide the manipulator with some of the best ways to get you to do what they want.

Fear of Being Alienated

No one wants to be alienated. They want to feel like they are a part of the group. They want to feel accepted as though they belong. This is never more apparent than when we see a newcomer. When someone is new to town, or to school, to work, or somewhere else, you will notice that they are trying to figure out how to join into the group and get them to accept them. They are worried that they are going to be alienated, and to avoid this, they will do everything in their powers to get others to like them and go along with them, and this is where the manipulator can come in and get what they want.

Newcomers who start to join a new manipulative group are usually going to receive a warm welcome—and they will form some new friendships that seem to be much more profound, and have a lot more commitment and meaning behind them compared to anything that they were able to experience in the past.

There are several reasons for this one. First, this gets the target to feel welcome and more indebted to the group, and the manipulator. They are thankful that they have these deep connections, and it is usually easier to get a friend to go along with something as compared to a stranger, so it works to the benefit of the manipulator as well. Add in that the target is scared to be alienated, then they are going to do what they can to keep the relationships going strong.

If any doubts end up arising in the future, these relationships are going to become a powerful tool to ensure they stay with the group. Even if they aren't completely convinced, the target will start to remember their outside world, the world that they had before joining this group, and it is going to seem cold and lonely. They will instead choose to stay with the group, even if there is some manipulation going on.

Fatigue

How well do you make decisions when you are tired? Do you find that you want to go to bed, and this makes you tired, irritable and very moody? Oftentimes, the decisions that you make are going to be questionable, and you may agree to do things that you would never have agreed to if you had gotten enough sleep.

This is another technique that the manipulator can use against their target. They know that their target isn't going to be able to make some significant decisions during this time, and they are going to use this to their advantage. They will make sure to find you when you are the most tired, and then make the requests that they want during this time.

Fatigue, as well as sleep deprivation, is going to result in anyone feeling tired, both mentally and physically. When the target is physically exhausted and less alert, they are going to find that it is hard to stand up against some of the persuasion that someone throws at them, especially if it is done by someone skilled in persuasion and manipulation.

You don't have to go very long before this power of persuasion can start to take effect. This is terrible news for the target, but good news for the manipulator. According to some research that has been explored in the Journal of Experimental Psychology, individuals who have not slept for 21 hours straight were more susceptible to suggestion.

Think about how many times you may have missed out on one night of sleep. If you are a parent, have stayed up too late working on a project for work or school, or ended up going out with some friends and staying out too late, you have quickly gone for just 21 hours without getting the sleep that you need— and sometimes, you may go even longer. However, with that short amount of time, it can be enough for you to not think in the manner that you should, and the manipulator can get what they want out of you.

Think about what would happen if you were able to go for a more extended period without sleep. If the manipulator could catch you after a few nights of the baby teething, or a few nights cramming for an exam, what would they be able to convince you of that you would never agree to in the past?

What the manipulator worked to create was a situation that was going to keep you awake. This is usually seen as something a bit more extreme, but it is possible that the manipulator will go through a process to isolate their target, and they may even work to make sure that this person isn't able to get the amount of sleep that they need. If they could limit the amount of sleep, maybe allowing the target to have only a few hours of sleep a night for a week, or keeping the target awake for 30 hours, think about what the manipulator would be able to get the target to agree to in the process.

Chapter 5: Personalities Likely to Manipulate

What Makes the Narcissist a Dangerous Manipulator?

It's not just arrogance and vanity that contribute to a narcissist's delusion of superiority—it's the grandiose idea that they are more important than everyone else around them that leads the narcissist to believe they are special enough to warrant getting anything that they want. They see themselves as being better than everyone else, and they only want to associate with those whom they deem to be on the same level as they are. What makes the narcissist such a dangerous type of manipulative personality (which is why it is part of the Dark Triad) is because they don't just believe they deserve respect and recognition—they demand it. They've created a skewed perception of reality in their mind in which they are the star of their show, and everyone else is merely a supporting player.

Anything and anyone that is perceived as a threat just waiting to burst the bubble of their fantasy world is going to be met with extreme reactions which could include defensiveness, warnings, and even outright rage. Since they have a constant need to be praised, admired, and recognized (also though they may have done nothing outstanding), maintaining a healthy relationship with a narcissist becomes nearly impossible. The connection is doomed to be one-sided from the start, a relationship where mutual benefit does not exist since the only one that stands to gain anything is the narcissist.

Since they genuinely believe they deserve to get anything they want because they're better than everyone else around them, they expect everyone to automatically bend over backward and comply with their every demand without question. To the narcissist, anyone who doesn't meet their requirements or go along with what they want is considered useless and invaluable. Should you be brave enough to deny their requests or even be so bold as to ask for a favor in return for the help you've given them, it won't take much for them to fly off the handle and react aggressively in anger, outrage or even emotionally torture you by subjecting you to the silent treatment.

The narcissist is a danger to your mental and emotional wellbeing for the simple reason that they have no regrets and will be more than willing to take advantage of exploit you for their gain without shame or remorse for their actions. This inflated sense of self-worth leads them to believe that they are entitled to treat you any way that they see fit, and they'll never see their actions as being wrong or immoral in any way.

In several ways, the narcissist has almost earned their spot in the Dark Triad, and one of the biggest reasons why is that they view everyone else around them as objects to be used. To the narcissist, you exist for no other purpose other than to serve their needs, and that is it. They will never stop to think twice about taking advantage of you, only to discard you when you no longer serve any useful purpose to them. They can be both malicious and oblivious at the same time, blinded mostly by their self of entitlement. They are incapable of thinking how their actions could have consequences on everyone else, even if you were to point it out to them, they'd dismiss and refuse to believe you.

The narcissist will demean you, bully you and belittle you if it means they're going to get their way. If they feel threatened by you or perceive you as trying to "push back" against them, they resort to putting you down to inflate their already inflated ego. In their mind, this is how they neutralize their "enemies," by stomping on them until they feel too insecure about rising and challenge them in any way. Threats, bullying, insults, shaming, dismissiveness, and ridicule are just some of the many tactics they will employ in an attempt to get you back in line and put you in your place.

Manipulators and Their Covert-Aggressive Personalities

When it comes to aggression, there are two categories they could fall into. They either resort to overt-aggression or covert-aggression. When someone is obvious, direct, and open in the manner with which they choose to stand up or fight back, that's over-aggression. This is a category the manipulator is unlikely to fall into since they never want anyone to know what they're really up to. No, a manipulator prefers to go with the second option, which is covert-aggression, a method which allows them to be deceptive, subtle, and underhanded enough to hide their true intentions. However, a very powerful manipulator will know how to use both traits and harness the combined power of both, avoiding any outright displays of overt-aggression while still being able to intimidate another enough to get them to do what you want. Covert-aggression is a manipulator's preferred mode of operation when it comes to interpersonal interaction.

Covert-aggression is not necessarily an act that is reserved for manipulators alone. Almost everyone has engaged in some form of covertly aggressive behavior now and then. Occasionally have to resort to covert-aggressive action for one reason or another does not mean you have a covert-aggressive type of personality. When you habitually repeat this type of behavior the way a manipulator does, then it becomes part of your personality. Manipulators with covert-aggressive characters rely on a steady diet of control, deception, and manipulation to keep them going. This tactic has become a part of who they are, and their preferred way of dealing with everyone else around them to get things done the way they want it to go.

For those who have never experienced it first-hand, they might have a hard time understanding why victims of manipulation have a hard time realizing what's going on, and why they fail to see that they're being taken advantage. It can be tempting to brush the victims off and assume that they're foolish for allowing themselves to be manipulated in that way. That is until you come to understand that there are excellent reasons why the victims fail to realize they're being manipulated until it's too late.

Chapter 6: NLP and Depression

If you're like millions of people in the world who struggle with depression, this is an essential chapter for you! Although depression can be treated and handled in several ways, Neuro-Linguistic Programming might be another option for you! You may have tried other options or strategies in the past, and maybe they haven't worked, or they haven't helped you in the way you've hoped. You may even be hoping to try a form of treatment that avoids and doesn't require medication. Whatever reason you have sought out this book, there is no doubt you will gain valuable information on the topic and how to use it in your specific way.

Reframing

The first strategy of discussion is called reframing. This means to see the situation in a different light or to put a different spin on it so you can view it differently! This strategy is intended to help you look at the more positive side of things, rather than any negative aspects. An example of this would be the following scenario: Imagine you have a son or daughter that often acts unruly. Always disagreeing and stating their strong opinion. For many, this may be frustrating, and you may view it as disrespectful or a negative personality trait on their part. However, when practicing reframing, you would instead want to realize that your son or daughter is independent and strong-minded in a right way and that this could be very helpful and beneficial to them in the future.

Maybe instead of being upset by this, you may want to think of it more positively and be happy about it. To help you out, even more, you can use a step-by-step process to help you change your thinking and get you more accustomed to reframing.

The first step you would want to practice is to identify your bad or unwanted behavior. This may be addictive sleeping, procrastinating, comfort eating, or sloppy time management skills. This will involve beginning brutally honest with yourself to admit what's wrong. Now, internally communicate with the part of the body that is associated with negative behavior. This is your way of mentally and verbally recognizing that one, there is a problem and, two, you're confronting it.

Next, choose a positive intention and reaction to the negative behavior. For example, if you think a friend is mad at you and your afraid you're going to get in a fight with them, instead of choosing the adverse reaction, like, getting defense and yelling at your friends, try to instead think about how you can act calm, cool and collected just in case there ends up being any confrontation. Step number four is to find three different approaches to a problem. Brainstorm different ways you could approach the situation and make sure they are all on positive rather than negative.

Now, evaluate these three different approaches and ask your subconscious to accept them. You will feel your body take the ideas when it feels like peace and calms about the plans. If your body and mind seem to reject the plans, reassess the three previous plans you just had, and then try this step again. Now, think ahead to how this new, learned behavior will affect you in future situations as well as relationships. Will the change be positive? Do your body and mind accept this behavior? Do you feel that this is the best course of action? How will this behavior affect your work and social life? These are all critical questions to be asking yourself at the end and final step of reframing.

Memory Manipulation

The next NLP strategy you can use to combat your depression is called memory manipulation. This strategy is all about a situation and how you view it based on your personality, beliefs, morals, and opinions. What is so interesting about this topic is that two different people, who witness the very same event or experience the very same situation, can have completely different viewpoints of it. This is because everyone, based on their personality, morals, and beliefs interprets the event or situation utterly different than the person standing right beside them.

In order to understand this strategy, let's attempt a little exercise. First, think about a significant memory that you feel a certain way about, but you wish you felt differently. You will want to choose a memory that there is still quite a bit of emotion attached to, so you may find that this memory is somewhat recent or of great importance to you. It also means that this memory is also one you feel discomforted and upset by and you, therefore; wish there had been a different outcome and lasting memory. Now, do your best to relive this memory. Go back into your mind and watch yourself within the memory.

Remember every single detail that you can; this includes sights, smells, location, the people (if any) that were there and any conversation that may have happened. Now, after remembering it one time through, remember it again but this time, put a border around it as you see it. It can be a border of anything—flowers, a solid color, food, rainbows, etc. Now, see if this changes how you're feeling about it. Now, try remembering it again, but this time, remember it and play it through in your head in black and white.

How do you feel now? Is memory better? Keep remembering your specific, chosen memory, and keep making these small changes until you feel an emotional difference behind the changes. Whatever makes you feel most positive and even happy, then follow that change. Now, you can begin to play around with the memory you have of the people in your mind as well. If you feel anger towards the person or people in your mind, try imagining them instead in a funny way. For example, you can imagine your boss as a giant marshmallow or your mother with the face of a cow. Try to find something that makes you laugh and thus, changes the emotion that goes with this memory. Finally, you can play around with the sounds you remember in specific memories to change how you remember them and the feelings surrounding them.

To do this, remember your chosen memory again and change the speed of the way people are talking. In the first round, make them speak fast. Does this make you laugh? Does it make you feel happier about the memory than you may have previously? Now, try to slow down the dialogue in your mind. How does this affect the way you feel about the mind now? In a third cycle, try making everyone's voices high pitched and squeaky. How does this version of the mind make you feel? Finally, in a fourth cycle, remember the memory and bring yourself through it but now make the voices inside of it deep. When the memory is like this, how do you feel about it? After four cycles of this, you should be able to tell which version of the memory makes you think the best. Hence, choose that version, keep it, and whenever it comes up again in the future, do your best to remember it in that specific version.

Collapsing Anchors

In another strategy, called collapsing anchors, you can alter anything that, when you first think of it, instantly fills you with negativity, anger, regret or unrest. To do this, you will want to try the following exercise. First, choose something that makes you feel negativity. For example, that fight you had with your co-worker last week. Now, hold up one of your hands, straight out in front of you. Imagine the memory or the person you chose right there in your hand. You want to remember the person or the memory so vividly that you see it there, sitting in your outstretched hand. You want to feel like the person or mind you chose is sitting in the palm of your hand.

Now, at the same time, stretch out your other hand. In this hand, imagine a ball of light that is filled with whatever makes you most happy in this world. This should be a memory, a feeling, a person, a hobby, or even a combination of these things. You want this ball and whatever you choose to put inside it, to fill you up and grow larger and larger and larger. Allow the happiness of it to overcome and fill you up. Allow the ball of joy to increase so large that it overtakes whatever or whoever you have put in your other hand. Now, in the future, when you remember that person or that event, train your mind to think instead of the massive ball of happiness and whatever was inside of it rather than the person or memory. If you find yourself struggling to imagine this, keep doing the exercise over and over until it becomes more comfortable and more successful.

Pattern Interrupt

Our last NLP strategy to tackle depression is called pattern interrupt, and it has a lot to do with self-talk and the way you speak to yourself. So much of depression stems from what you do to yourself (including the way you talk to yourself) instead of what happens to you. Changing your mindset and how you speak to yourself can help you in massive ways if you're struggling with depression. An example of this strategy would be to run through a typical conversation you have with yourself daily.

Chapter 7: NLP and Anxiety

There is a possibility that if you have sought out this book, you may be having some struggles or frustrations with anxiety. If you have these struggles, you're not alone! Thirty-three percent of the population will develop some sort of anxiety disorder within their lifetimes, and, furthermore, nearly the same amount will have complaints about their doctor and his or her method of treatment. Hence, if you're looking for an alternative option, look no further!

First, it's essential to understand just what is causing your anxiety. Your anxiety is based on something you're afraid of and its consequences. For example, if you have social anxiety, you might be frightened of what possible bad things can happen to you when you're in a social environment. Another important aspect of your anxiety that is important to understand is that although there probably are simple solutions to whatever your fear may be, you instead choose to think of grandiose solutions that are entirely unrealistic.

Reframing Your Anxiety and Its Symptoms

Your very first technique when it comes to anxiety is to reframe your anxiety and the symptoms you're experiencing. To do this, picture yourself having a typical bout of anxiety and what that looks like for you. For example, you have anxiety when your boyfriend or husband is late coming home. You've arrived home, it gets late, he isn't home yet, he hasn't called, and you begin having anxiety thinking about where he might be, what he might be doing, who he might be with—and you lead yourself to believe absurd ideas, like he is never coming home again, and he is probably cheating on you.

There are a few factors here. First, you need to agree and come to terms with the fact that you have created the anxiety and your panic. You're the one who got all worked up and began telling yourself these things. Is there or was there ever any real, factual proof for any of your thoughts? Chances are, the answer is no. If so, you have just identified your first problem. Now, think of your strategy. What thought process led you to believe these things? What did you tell yourself? Are these things grounded in facts? Or, are you making things up and jumping to conclusions? Think about your train of thought during your anxiety and identify the good and the bad.

Furthermore, ask yourself if you could explain this train of thought to someone else. If you can, you have now identified another problem. This is because you are so sure of these things that are causing you anxiety that you have convinced yourself so much that you could also convince another person. That's how deeply you have overreacted. It's important to identify this harmful process. Next, think about this same situation that is causing you anxiety and talk about it out loud but, this time, as if you're watching someone else do it.

Does this seem realistic and like a normal thought process? Chances are, your answer is no. Now, you have fully realized, from many points of view, why this thought process that is causing your anxiety is causing you so much frustration and negativity. You now need to teach yourself to choose a different thought process. You can do this by self-talking yourself through different scenarios and choosing positive trains of thought rather than negative.

Accessing Resources and Accessing Solutions

The next technique you can use to tackle your anxiety problems is by doing something called accessing resources and accessing solutions. Oftentimes, there are events or certain things in your life that trigger your anxiety. This technique focuses on that trigger and helps you to cope with how this trigger and the situation makes you feel as well as how you can solve this. First, you need to identify your problem and its trigger.

For example, maybe at work, when your boss speaks to you in a very short way, it creates anxiety for you because you feel like he or she is angry at you or treating you unfairly. Now that you've pinpointed the problem, it's time to tackle it. You can do this by asking yourself a series of questions. For example, "What do you want to achieve by solving this problem?" "What do you want to happen to make you feel relieved?" "How will you know this problem is solved?" or "If and when this problem is solved, how and what will you feel?" Answer these questions honestly, and reflect on the answers.

You may start to realize that you've answered quite a few questions for yourself, especially as to how you can solve your problem just by exploring it with those questions. Next, you're going to ask yourself another series of questions. This time, you want to think about times when the problem that leads to your anxiety isn't happening.

Then, ask yourself the following questions: "What are the times when you feel the problem isn't as bad or doesn't exist at all?" What were you doing at that time? Were you doing anything differently than you usually do or anything out of the ordinary? You may realize that with these questions, your eyes are opened to times when your anxiety is lessened and maybe even nonexistent. If you find yourself realizing this, focus on your behavior at this time and how you can teach yourself to have that behavior more consistently.

However, if you find that this second set of questions doesn't apply to you, move onto one last set of what is referred to as "miracle questions." For example: "Imagine, one night, as your sleeping deeply, that the problem or problems that cause your anxiety have magically or by some miracle has been solved. You have no idea how this problem was solved, as you were deep asleep but when you wake up, how do you know the problem or problems have been solved? What's different? What gives it away? This may give you some answers to how you need to change your train of thought or attitude to make this change happen and avoid your anxiety.

Trance and Utilizing Relaxation Anchors

Another technique you can use is trance, as well as learning to utilize relaxation anchors. The very first way to do this is to teach and train yourself to stop flexing and tightening certain muscle groups that cause you to be tenser and thus more anxious. Some of these vital muscle groups might be your jawline, the muscles in your forehead and clenching your hands. If you find yourself growing anxious or experiencing the problems you usually do when your anxiety presents itself, take a second to check these muscle groups. Are they flexed and tightened? If so, take a second to fix this and then see how you feel!

You may not even realize how big of a difference this may make in your anxiety levels! Next, pay attention and focus on you're out breathing rather than when you breathe in. When your body experiences anxiousness, it's natural to quicken and tense up your inward breathing movements. Instead of allowing this to happen, focus on breathing out in a calm, relaxing way. This may help to calm you down if you're experiencing anxiety. Lastly, you want to focus on the mental imagery you have in your head.

As humans, we spend a large portion communicating with ourselves inside our heads. This communication includes mental imagery, and oftentimes, people who experience anxiety on different levels have negative mental images that they are feeding and creating for themselves. Train yourself and your mind to avoid this. To do this, you can start training yourself on a daily basis.

For example, throughout your day, keep track and be aware of what mental images are coming into your mind. When you experience a negative one, immediately put a stop to it and replace it with a positive one. This will take quite a bit of self-talk and self-discipline, but if you commit to it and persevere, you will be surprised and pleased with just how much of your anxiety and thinking you can change!

Anchoring

Finally, one last technique you can use for any anxiety you're experiencing in your life is through something called anchoring. This is also similar to classical conditioning. The entire point of this technique involves finding what external cue is triggering an internal response and learning to change this external cue to change your response.

For example, you have a severe fear of monkeys, and when you see monkeys, you become internally scared and frightened. This triggers your anxiety. In order to change this behavior, you want to train yourself to make a link between the external cue and the internal emotion. To do this, you want to associate whatever the cue may probably be with something positive rather than negative.

Hence, for example, if you have a fear of monkeys, you would want to train your mind to associate the sight of monkeys with something you really love, for example, your children or your favorite memory instead of a stream of terrifying made up outcomes as to what might happen when you come in contact with monkeys. Or, you can even choose an object to change the emotional attachment to the cue. For example, when you see the picture of monkeys, you can choose an object that you greatly connect with or something that means a lot to you and concentrate on that to avoid the negative emotion that triggers your anxiety.

You can even bring this object with you to physically look at it and focus on it instead of focusing on the emotions of fear, anger, or sadness. One other way you can use anchoring is through sound association. Just as with the last previous options, you can think of a sound that means a lot to you or that you associate many happy memories with and use that to help curb the emotions that trigger your anxiety. For example, when you see monkeys or pictures of monkeys, you can try to think of the sound of your grandfather's voice or the sound of your baby laughing.

You can train your brain to think of these things instead of fear and thus, turn your upsetting emotions into happy ones. Finally, the last tool you can use for anchoring is the idea of an important relationship to combat any negative feelings. When you see the cue to whatever causes the trigger, you want to train your mind to think of the positive, happy relationship you have chosen instead of your negative emotions.

Chapter 8: Subliminal Persuasion

Understanding the Subconscious Mind

Subliminal persuasion is a term that is found in advertising quite a bit. It can often be associated with the idea of tricking someone into picking up a message, but oftentimes, the person doesn't realize that they are picking up that message. This kind of persuasion is done on a level that it is hard for the victim to pick up on how it is being done quickly.

This is just another of the tactics of manipulation that many people are going to use on those around them. Subliminal persuasion might not be seen as something as harmful or invasive as the other topics that we have discussed in this guidebook, but it is still something that can influence the victim, often without the victim even being aware of it, which makes it dangerous. Also, compared to the other forms of manipulation that we have talked about in this book, subliminal persuasion is often the hardest of them to detect, which makes it the hardest to combat.

The idea that comes with this subliminal persuasion is that it can send out influences to others, influences that stay below the detectable conscious human level. Those who are being manipulated in this manner aren't going to realize what is going on until it is too late. In some cases of manipulation, one can recognize that it is happening at that time. But for the most part, those who are manipulated in this manner can go for years before even realizing that this has happened.

How Does the Subconscious Mind Work?

There are two parts of the brain, the conscious mind, and the subconscious mind. Our subconscious mind is going to work the hardest out of the two. This part is never going to shut down, even when we sleep, and it is always on the lookout for what kind of decisions we need to make. Depending on the situation, it will make these decisions before we even realize what is going on.

Even when we are resting and letting our conscious mind take a break, the subconscious is putting on various movies for us to look over, in the form of dreams. This part of the brain has so much information available to it that it can create things like dreams, daydreams, delusions, and other forms of dissociation in a way to process all that it knows.

It is impressive how limitless our brains are. There might be several things we can know, but it hasn't been found yet. So far, researchers have only been able to make assumptions on how now they think that the brain can go. And even though we can pack information into the brain all day long, all without feeling like we know too much, many of us are happy working with the knowledge that we already have.

It is incredible how powerful our subconscious mind is. It is going to consume an estimated 95 percent of our brain, but we don't necessarily have full control over it. This part of our mind is often believed to be the reason why we develop specific fears, or why some people have certain addictions. If you had ever had a time when you had the emotion or a thought, but you weren't sure why you were having these, that is probably because the subconscious sent it your way for one reason or another.

Your subconscious mind is always working, no matter how much you may have been slacking off before. Remember that one time that you decided to stay up all night to finish a test or a project? You may not specifically be able to recollect that night, but your subconscious sure can. It's what's reminding you to get the work done on time, rather than procrastinating again so that you won't have to pull an all-nighter and deal with that pain and worry ever again.

You will find, if you delve deep enough and explore enough, that the key to many of our known issues is going to lie directly in our subconscious. Why might someone think that dogs are scary? If they took a look into the subconscious mind, the most likely would see that they internalized something dark in their past that in turn made them more fearful about dogs.

Even though we are learning more and more about our subconscious mind each day, there is still so much that we don't know. And it is possible that we will never fully understand or learn about the subconscious or how it works. But this certainly doesn't mean that we shouldn't give it a try. The more that we can understand how the brain works, on all levels, the better we will get when it's time to fix it in the long run.

The subconscious mind is going to play an important role when it comes to affecting the way that you behave, in shaping the way that your personality will be, and many other aspects of your life. Many people don't understand how the subconscious mind is going to work, or what kinds of mechanisms need to be in place to govern its operation.

To get a better understanding of how this part of the mind works, you can remember that it is going to handle all of the things that we are not necessarily conscious about at any given time. For example, you may have a fear of public speaking. And this fear could come from the unconscious belief that you are unattractive and that people are going to make fun of you when you get up to speak. While you may not be aware of that belief at all, it is still going to have a significant effect on the way that you behave, and on how well you do with the public speaking.

The subconscious mind can be thought of like a big bank of memories, one that is going to store not just these memories, but also your experiences and your beliefs. This information is all going to be stored there, even though it might take some effort to bring it back out again. Even though we may not realize it is there, we are going to find that it can affect our actions and our behavior in different situations. Hence, if you lack self-confidence in yourself because there are some beliefs in your subconscious mind, then you may find that when you are around others, you feel anxious. This is because your mind has some information, information that is most likely false, that made you believe that you were in danger, even though there is no danger present around you.

You have to be very careful about this subconscious mind. It not only gets to control your behavior, but it can also affect the perception of events and how you look at the world around you. If in the previous case, you saw that two people are nearby and who smiled back at you while looking at you, then you might fall into the mistaken belief that they are trying to make fun of you.

Always remember that the mind is going to feed you more of what you focus on. Because you already had that false belief about yourself, you would start to look around to see if there is some proof for this. And you are going to be able to find it if you look hard enough. The good news is that you can work with this part of the mind if you choose. Many of us don't understand how this part of the mind works. This is why many of us will set a goal and assume that we will be able to reach them overnight. But because of some of the habits that we have formed throughout the years, and because of how our subconscious mind is set up.

It is tough for the subconscious to accept a brand new belief, especially if it is one that contradicts an opinion that is already there. This means that it can be tough for you to accept that you are a confident person if you have spent years believing that you had no confidence and that no one wanted to be with you.

This doesn't mean that all hope is lost. Otherwise, the manipulator wouldn't waste their time on anyone older than three who had lots of thoughts in their subconscious mind already. There are a few steps that you can take to make this part of the brain work for you, including:

i.   Change the beliefs that are held in your subconscious mind by using some actions. If you want to change the beliefs that you have, such as "I am not good at math," then you must make sure that you put this into action. Maybe you can ignore that thought and study hard so that you start getting good grades in math. Then, the subconscious mind will begin to see that you are pretty good at math, and these beliefs will begin to change.

ii. Do go against these beliefs: Don't use any affirmations that don't make sense to your subconscious mind. These may sound great, but if they go against some powerful beliefs, then you may need to work with something else to get them to work.

iii.   Remember that your subconscious is not going to do magic for you. Some people believe that their subconscious can do some extraordinary things. For example, they may think that they can use this part of the brain to lose weight while they still get to eat anything that they want. But these kinds of thoughts show that these people don't know how the subconscious mind works at all.

iv.   Now, you can work with this part of the mind to lose weight, but you have to put in some action, rather than just assuming the mind is going to do it on its own. For example, you could modify some of your beliefs, do start working out more, and be careful with the food you eat in order to lose weight.

Persuasion

How is a manipulator going to get people to think and behave differently? There are many subtle ways that they can use to press their agenda without turning the victim off or even letting them realize what is going on. In the area of persuasion, there are six main principles, including what we talked about earlier, and will include the following:

a) Reciprocity

b) Consistency and commitment

c) Social proof

d) Authority

e) Likability

f) Scarcity

While persuasion is a type of science, it can also be seen as an art. If a person pushes too hard, then they are going to come off as being aggressive. But the manipulator is going to be able to do the right balance between using persuasion without becoming aggressive so no red flags will come up. They will befriend the other person, talk with them, and make sure that the two are on the same page as much as possible. Then, they will start to use some of the tactics of persuasion to gain control over the other person, and get the power that they want.

The Psychology of Persuasion

When you hear the word persuasion, what do you think about first? Some may think about advertising messages that they see all the time, the ones that focus on trying to get the viewer to choose a particular product or go after a political candidate.

Persuasion is a mighty force that we are going to see in our daily life, and it does have a level of influence on society as a whole, as well as on the individual. Mass media, legal decisions, news, politics, advertising, and more are all going to be influenced by the power of persuasion and that same persuasion is going to affect us as well.

Many people believe that they are immune to persuasion. They think that they can see through any sales pitch that comes their way, and have a good comprehension about what the truth is in any given situation. This might be true some of the time, but there are so many different types of persuasion, and they aren't all going to be a push a salesman who wants to sell you something or even a commercial on the television. You will find that persuasion can be subtle. And it can come from people we are close to, ones we wouldn't expect at all. The way that we are going to respond to these influences is going to depend on our background, along with many other factors.

When most people think about persuasion, they are going to focus on some of the negative examples of it. This is the way that a manipulator would try to use persuasion. But there are times when belief can be used in more of a positive way. For example, if you have ever seen a public service campaign that urged people to stop smoking, or to recycle, then you have seen an example of positive persuasion.

So this brings up the question, what is persuasion? According to Perloff in 2003, persuasion is "a symbolic process in which communicators try to convince other people to change their attitudes or behaviors regarding an issue through the transmission of a message in an atmosphere of free choice."

Always remember that no matter how intense the persuasion is, the victim does get a choice in how they act. The manipulator may work to take away this choice or make it seem like there aren't any choices, but there is still that freedom of the choice present. There are a few key elements that come into play when we are talking about persuasion. These are going to include:

1) Persuasion is something symbolic. It is going to use a variety of features, including sounds, images, words, and more.

2) Persuasion is going to involve a deliberate attempt by one person to influence another person or a group of people.

3) Self-persuasion is key. The person is always going to have the freedom to make a choice, and they will never be coerced.

4) Methods of transmitting persuasive messages can occur in many different ways. This can include options that are nonverbal and verbal, as well as through face to face, internet, radio, television, and more communication options.

What Is Subliminal Persuasion?

Subliminal persuasion is going to be the technique of convincing your target, or your group of goals, to do something, without them knowing. There isn't going to be any outward suggesting of the idea, and often the victim isn't going to realize that you were trying to influence them at all. It is one of the types of persuasion that manipulators and others can use, and it is going to use words, along with some gestures, to get ahold of different people. Hence, you may find things like smiling, use of the head, eye expression, and more being used, both positively and negatively. It is a powerful technique, but often a challenging technique, that not only uses words, but uses the meaning behind the words, and body language, to ensure that the victim does what the manipulator wants.

In our modern world, the techniques that are used for subliminal persuasion are going to be powerful weapons that can help you get ahead. They can help you to manipulate others, or even gain an advantage in a market where there is a lot of competition, and you need to stay ahead of the game. According to some experts in the field of marketing and persuasion, many people choose subliminal advertising because it is more effective. As they say, "Persuasion that looks like persuasion isn't persuasive anymore."

Even a manipulator can use this information to help them take control of the victim. If the persuasion that they use is too apparent, then the victim is just going to walk away. We see so many examples of persuasion in our daily lives that it is easy to recognize the more apparent signs and stay away from them if we don't want to purchase something or do something. If a manipulator comes at their victim with a big sales pitch, lots of bright flashing lights, and other apparent techniques of persuasion, then they will get nowhere. The victim is smart enough to recognize these signs, and they will get away from the manipulator, and the manipulator—and this is where subliminal persuasion can come in.

Every time that the manipulator communicates with their victim, they are going to be very careful about the nonverbal signs that they are sending out as well. While they still have to say words (your victim is going to notice if you stand around sending out nonverbal cues and never talking), the manipulator is going to try and send out other messages and extra persuasion through the body language and the nonverbal cues that they are sending out as well.

Since subliminal persuasion is going to deal with the feelings that the victim has, there is going to be some subconscious element in this kind of persuasion. As a manipulation or another type of person who needs to use persuasion, you will provide the victim's mind with some feelings of enthusiasm and comfort about doing a given task. Those thoughts and emotions are going to be sent out to the subconscious mind, but then we have to take to the logical mind to. You can then talk to this part of the mind by discussing the things that are rational about the choice.

Now, there are going to be a few subliminal factors that are going to influence whether the manipulator is going to be believable. For instance, the way that the manipulator does dress is going to be a factor. They are going to make sure that the victim sees the manipulator at their very best. They will dress nicely, make sure that their appearance is kept up, and always look like they are doing well. Even when they are trying to play the victim and say that they are hurt or dealing with an illness, your manipulator will still dress nice.

The reason for this is the likeability factor that we talked about before. We are programmed to be more likely to help out someone with a beautiful appearance, someone who is well-groomed, compared to someone who is not. If the manipulator wants to exploit this factor, then they are going to take some extra precautions with their appearance.

There can also be a level of subliminal persuasion that is used in the language of the manipulator as they ask for a favor. There is a lot of truth in the idea of "it's not what you say, but how you say it." The manipulator isn't going to say anything that is too out there, because this is something that may raise some flags with their victim. But the way they use their words will make a difference, and usually gets them what they want.

The way that the manipulator will use their inflections and intonations will also have a bearing on the meaning of what you say. If you see a sentence like "I can't promise you that price," you may assume that it has just one meaning, and that is it. But depending on the way that the manipulator, or salesperson, uses it, there may be a few different meanings. Take a look at some of the examples below to see what we mean here:

a) I can't promise you that price. This one can infer that one person can't do it, but maybe there is someone else who can offer that price.

b) I can't promise you that price. This one is going to infer that there is just no way that the person is going to get that price.

c) I can't promise you that price. This one is going to infer that there isn't a guarantee, but that the manipulator might be able to do them a "favor' and get that price.

d) I can't promise you that price. This one is going to infer that the manipulator isn't willing to get you that price, but maybe they will guarantee that price to someone else.

e) I can't guarantee you that price. This one infers that the manipulator is going to see what they can do. They may not be able to offer precisely that, but they could still get you something good.

f)   I can't promise you that price. This one is going to infer that they will still be able to guarantee you something, even if the price point doesn't fall in the desired spot.

The meaning of statements is a great way to utilize the ideas of subliminal persuasion. And there can be so many different meanings based on the words that the manipulator or any other person decides to emphasize. And it is sometimes such a subtle process, that we can hear the sentence and infer the meaning, without even realizing what is going on.

Think about the intonation that you can use when you say a specific sentence, and then imagine the power that goes behind those words based on what a manipulator would be able to use with them as well. There are about three choices that come with intonation and the way that it can change up the meaning of the whole sentence. As we go through and say something, the three ways to finish up that sentence would include:

a)   A downward, which would mean that the intonation is a deeper voice

b)   A voice intonation that doesn't change at all

c)   An intonation that goes up

Different Ways That You Are Persuaded Subliminally (And You Don't Even Realize It!)

Whether you feel comfortable with the idea or not, you may be subliminally persuaded in one way or another. For example, if someone has ever used a form of passive-aggressive behavior on you, then they have tried to use this kind of persuasion on you as well. For example, your mother could comment how they saw someone at the store that they hadn't seen for some time, and then they make a snide comment about the weight of that person, in a confident tone.

The reason that the mother was doing this could be a subliminal message about how that mother feels about the weight of her daughter. The persuasion then is that the perception of that daughter is going to be altered. For example, the daughter may feel like she isn't meeting the standards of beauty that her mother has. And as a result, the daughter could try to alter her life, choosing to stay away from the mother to avoid these comments and not feel bad or try to work and lose weight if possible.

This is such a tricky tactic of persuasion, one of the hardest to fight off out of them all. Those who are using this kind of persuasion are often going to be so lost in their delusions, ones that no one else is going to share, and they are never able to recover. Of course, they are never going to admit that they are using these manipulation tactics, and the victim will need to remove themselves from the situation, or they will be stuck in the cycle forever.

Asking for More

One method that someone who is a subliminal persuader will use to get something from others is to start by asking for more than they need in the end. Perhaps that person needs to have $5000, but they know that is a significant amount to ask someone for, especially right from the beginning. Hence, instead of starting with that amount, they are going to ask for one that is much higher. This is done to kind of shock the victim into thinking the lower amount is more reasonable, and they are more likely to give in to the request.

For example, if the manipulator needs $5000, they may ask for $12,000. They know that the second amount is going to be a tremendous amount of money and that there is no way that the person is going to give them that amount. The victim may feel bad because they aren't able to provide that amount, and they may think that the manipulator needs that large of an amount. To try and still help out, even though it is a large sum of money, the victim may offer to give half the amount, say $6000, or another amount, to see if that will help.

In this one, the victim has been tricked. They give the $6000 because they at least feel in this situation that they have given something to the manipulator and that they are helping out in some manner. They may even feel bad for not being able to offer the original amount that was requested. But the manipulator walks away happy. They walked away from this with $6000, even though they only needed $5000, and they won in the end.

The person who was the victim of this subliminal persuasion may feel guilty at the end of this conversation because they weren't able to give more, and they weren't able to help out for the full amount. Even though that person already asked for something once, the manipulator can keep on coming back because their victim will feel like they hadn't given enough the first time. Or, since they helped in the past, they may feel obligated to keep up with this pattern and offer help again.

Doing Favors

Someone who is using subliminal persuasion on another person may first choose to ask for a favor. With manipulation, it is more of a demand or a blatant telling of what the victim needs to do. But the persuader will ask for the favor so that there is an illusion that they need some help that only the victim can provide. The victim is going to feel like they should help out because they may have some need to care for others, and they may feel good about themselves for doing a favor for someone else.

In some cases, the manipulator may do a favor for the other person first. This helps the victim feel like since they had gotten help. First, they need to return the favor, and they become indebted to the manipulator—but with the subliminal persuasion, the manipulator is just going to cut to the chase and will focus on appearing like they need help with something.

Those who are the victim in these cases may feel like they are someone special, just because they get the privilege of helping this other person out. They may feel good about themselves like they had some value because they were able to help someone else. Of course, the manipulator is the one in control of that situation, and they are taking advantage of the need to care in the victim to their advantage they will get what they wanted from the victim, even though the victim is going to feel good about doing the favor.

This is a technique that can be seen with bosses in many cases. They may pick out a member who is on their team to a unique position, which makes that individual feel like they are superior and exceptional. In reality, the tasks that this person is given are ones that anyone can do, but the boss didn't want to handle them, so the boss handed them off to this employee.

If you think that someone is trying to use subliminal persuasion on you, it may be a good idea for you to ask that person whether they can go without that favor, or if they can do it for themselves. You always have to consider why they are asking you to do that task. What is the personal gain that they are going to get when you do the work? This can help you figure out if the intentions of the other person are pure or not.

Being Flattered

Flattery can be a great thing, but it is something that can be used against the victim when the manipulator gets to work. The manipulator will believe that if they can build up their victim, and if they can make that victim feel good about themselves, then they can get what they want out of that person.

You can see how well flattery works when you watch young children use this technique. Children often learn how to use flattery at an early age in an attempt to get people to do what they want. They already understand that using their charm can lead to a lot of happiness in other people, which will lead them to do things for the manipulator.

It isn't just something that younger children will use. Many adults will work on flattery as a form of subliminal persuasion. For example, how often have we heard of a young woman who uses flattery for an older man, one who isn't that good looking, but who has a lot of money and could make her life more comfortable? That is something that can occur in abuse as well. The abuser gets into a pattern of building up the significant other a bunch, and then later when it works for them, they are going to tear this person down and be the one in control of the situation again.

You will find that people are much more willing to do something for the manipulator when there is flattery involved. The flattery, even if it is shallow or also if it is from someone we don't know well, makes us feel good. It makes us feel smarter, prettier, stronger, and more like. This can all come together and makes us feel like we owe something to the person who took the time to flatter us, and then the manipulator has the upper hand and can use that to their advantage over us.

Choosing the Right Time to Ask for Something

Those who are going to be using subliminal persuasion are going to make sure that they calculate out the right time to ask for something. They won't just focus on who to go after as a victim. They are also going to put in some effort into deciding when it is the right time to ask the victim to help with the favor to make sure the answer is going to be a yes.

There are a lot of times when the manipulator can choose to ask you for a favor. But it will never be at a time when you are at your best. They won't ask you when you are having a good day, or when you are well-rested and happy or ready to think through the answers that you give. This is when ordinary people would ask because they want to get an appropriate response from you.

But remember that the manipulator wants to get the answer that benefits them. And they often know that you will turn them down if you are alert enough to catch on to what they are asking for This is why you must be careful about requests for favors or help when you are tired, or even times when you are in a good mood. The manipulator is going to spend some time looking for these times and then using them to their advantage when they ask you for some favors.

The manipulator who is using subliminal persuasion is going to wait until their victim is at the right place. They will choose a time when you are tired, or even when you are a perfect mood. They are patient, and they will make sure that they wait until the right time to ask you for something The manipulators want to make sure that their victim is going to say yes, and they will wait until that time comes.

Someone who is trying to subliminally persuade you will also try to ask for favors when both of you are in public settings. They believe that this is going to give them the upper hand of the situation. They like to do this because it can take away the chance for a confrontation that is going to be uncomfortable and unfavorable for them.

In some instances, they will ask for the favor when you are in front of your family and friends. That makes it so that the person who is the victim feel like they should do the support because it allows them to show off how generous they are to other people. And that is why this kind of persuasion can be so difficult to detect in some cases.

When the victim can help, they are going to feel good about themselves. They can see what the other person needs, and then they will step in and offer to help in some way. They can feel good about themselves, and they can sometimes look good in front of the other people who are important to them, and the manipulator gets to leave with exactly what they wanted because the victim followed the plan.

Conclusion

The next step is to make sure that you use these techniques to protect yourself against manipulation, persuasion, and NLP in your daily life. There are always people trying to persuade you and manipulate you—and while some of these are going to do so in a beneficial way that can help not only them but also you, most individuals who use manipulation are only interested in getting what they want and aren't concerned about how it affects you at all.

This guidebook has spent some time taking a look at manipulation and persuasion, as well as how the victim can often get stuck in this kind of cycle, thus providing benefits to the manipulator even though it may not be suitable for them, without even realizing what is going on. We then looked at some of the ways to recognize what is going on and to know the signs and break free so that the victim can live the life that they want, free from the manipulator.

When you are ready to learn more about the world of dark psychology, manipulation, persuasion, and NLP tactics, make sure to read this guidebook to help you get started. Sometimes, the act of manipulation can occur right in front of us, and we don't even know it. Why? It's because we miss the signs, signals, and body language cues that indicate that there might be more to that person than meets the eye. We have all, in one way or another, been guilty of manipulation—or we've been the victim of a manipulator's underhanded tactics. There are many aspects that build manipulation: persuasive words, body language, and tone of voice are all channels to convey or communicate manipulative messages. However, is manipulation harmful—or is it a case of a little harmless persuasion that won't hurt anyone? Why is manipulation wrong, and what if it is done for the good of the one manipulated? The book will play a key role in helping you understand the dark psychology of the human mind, as well as how to identify the subtle body language signals all around you!

Book Description

Has it come to your realization that all people have the ability to dupe others using manipulative techniques and can as well get tricked by others using many secrets of dark psychology?

Every person has the ability to victimize other people by preying on them. Whereas many restrain from this tendency, there are those who act on these instincts. Dark Psychology aims to identify such perceptions and thoughts that cause humans to be predatory. This book tries to explain Dark Psychology techniques that are used by people to influence, manipulate, and coerce others to get whatsoever they want. Dark Psychology is a science and art of mind control and manipulation. For so many years now, the concept of mind control has existed, and people have shown both fear and fascination of what would take place if an individual would control their thoughts and minds and lead them to do things that are against their wish and will. There have been conspiracy theories on how government officials, as well as other influential persons, use their talents and capacities to control actions of the minorities and small groups.

Inside the book, you will come across interesting topics such as:

- Neuro-Linguistic Programming and mind map

- Understanding the dark triad

- Manipulation and behavior conversion

- Mind control techniques

- Personalities likely to manipulate

- NLP and depression

- NLP and anxiety

- Subliminal persuasion

Each of the mind control tactics works in a different way. Brainwashing works to convince the subject to change their whole identity with the use of isolation and shaming, as well as to eventually offer a way to feel better that conforms to the new desired identity. Hypnosis allows the subject to enter a new altered state of mind where they will be more likely to be perceptive and open to new ideas. On the other hand, manipulation and deception will alter the current thought process of the subject using subterfuge as a primary tactic, while persuasion involves influencing a person's beliefs, attitudes, intentions, motivations, or behaviors.

In the modern world, dark psychology is among the most powerful forces used by the most influential people to manipulate others. People who are uneducated and uninformed are in the danger of having it used against them. Do not run the risks; this book will help you understand the secrets of dark psychology widely and in a manner that will assist you to overcome any tactics employed by the manipulator.

www.ingramcontent.com/pod-product-compliance
Lightning Source LLC
Chambersburg PA
CBHW072008150726
47999CB00002B/551